Praise for
Ally Hilfiger and

"It's riveting."

—Kathie Lee Gifford, *TODAY*

"BITE ME is a must-read. It is riveting, personal, and well written. Its spiritual message is powerful and inspirational. With love all things are possible."

—Russell Simmons

"This book will be very important at a time that Lyme disease meets NIH's eight characteristics of a worldwide pandemic. Thank you, sweet Ally, for daring to share your inspiring journey of strength, hope, and everyday determination to get well."

—Yolanda Hadid

"BITE ME is captivating. Ally recounts her experience battling misdiagnosis and a debilitating tormentor with a humor and power that can inspire us all. She gives a voice to others who are struggling."

—Georgia May Jagger

"Reading Ally's struggle of dealing with the debilitating effects of Lyme disease is a total inspiration. Her cheerful strength of will and determination to rise above the exhausting days of not knowing the way out proves once again that the human spirit can prevail in the most strenuous of circumstances."

—Bryan Adams

"A fascinating look at a disease that is often misdiagnosed and costs many people their sanity and lives. BITE ME is a story of courage. I highly recommend it." —Thalía Mottola

"An honest and poignant memoir…heartbreaking and heart-warming, Hilfiger's prose is ultimately helpful and hopeful." —*Hamptons Magazine*

"Brutally honest and raw, [Ally] opens up completely, inviting readers to see how dark and dramatic things became…Her advice? Keep fighting no matter how bad and challenging the struggle." —*BELLA New York Magazine*

"BITE ME is humorous and suspenseful, and it holds your attention to the very last page. This is a story that will inspire you." —Tommy Mottola

"After a tick bite at age seven, Ally Hilfiger started experiencing serious health issues, but her test for Lyme disease was inconclusive. And so began years of misdiagnoses, from growing pains to ADD to rheumatoid arthritis to MS to fibromyalgia—until she was finally diagnosed correctly at nineteen. Hilfiger, now thirty-one, chronicles her battle…Here, she talks desperation, healing, and a will to change the world." —*Marie Claire* bite me

bite

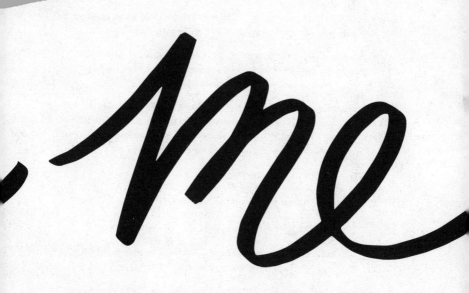

me

How Lyme Disease Stole My Childhood,

Made Me Crazy, and Almost Killed Me

ALLY HILFIGER

Foreword by TOMMY HILFIGER

CENTER
STREET

NEW YORK   BOSTON   NASHVILLE

Center Street
Hachette Book Group
1290 Avenue of the Americas, New York, NY 10104
centerstreet.com
twitter.com/centerstreet

Originally published in hardcover and ebook by Center Street in May 2016.
First Trade Edition: March 2017

Center Street is a division of Hachette Book Group, Inc. The Center Street name and logo are trademarks of Hachette Book Group, Inc.

The publisher is not responsible for websites (or their content) that are not owned by the publisher.

The Hachette Speakers Bureau provides a wide range of authors for speaking events. To find out more, go to www.HachetteSpeakersBureau.com or call (866) 376-6591.

Book design by Timothy Shaner, NightandDayDesign.biz.

Library of Congress Control Number: 2016934147

ISBNs: 978-1-4555-6705-8 (trade pbk.), 978-1-4555-6707-2 (ebook)

Printed in the United States of America

LSC-C

10 9 8 7 6 5 4 3 2 1

For my daughter, Harley. The hope of you was the reason to keep fighting. You are the light of my life.

contents

PART THREE

foreword

I remember it clearly: holding my baby girl Ally in the cab heading home from New York University Medical Center, where she was born, and freaking out every time the taxi hit a bump. I knew then that I would do anything to keep this child from harm.

As a young child, Ally was the most vivacious, outgoing, and fun little girl. We'd play outside in the leaves in the backyard or go hiking in the woods or collect seashells on the beach.

She was an incredibly social child, and would talk to anyone, especially those we would encounter on our travels, be it a cabdriver or a prince. I come from a big family, with eight brothers and sisters, and Ally fit right in. She carries the torch of the big love and big personalities of my clan.

She was also an old soul as a child. We would have long conversations about life, which she understood from a sophisticated angle from a very young age. I was pleasantly surprised every time I had a conversation with her. She'd ask the most intelligent questions and many times know the answer before she asked it—she would ask a question as a confirmation.

For a time, I was convinced she was going to be an actress on Broadway or in movies. She has a great singing voice, and is a gifted mimic. I think she got her social nature and talent for impersonations from me (I always wanted to be an actor), but she is incredibly creative, and has always had a great sense of style, which, along with her talent as an artist, she got from her mom, Susie.

There is an old saying that you are only as happy as your children, and when I began to see my daughter in pain I was in pain. From the time she was ten or so, we went to doctor after doctor and yet couldn't find out what was wrong. It was difficult to endure. I wished it were happening to me instead of my sweet, little girl. I wanted to believe that at some point we would find a cure or a way to help her heal from the pain that seem to get worse, but instead the medical community continued to misdiagnose my daughter. I felt helpless and, to be honest, even hopeless at times.

For Ally things went from bad to worse. In her late teens, she experienced a psychotic episode that lasted for several days. Leading up to it, I knew she was not herself. I also knew her self-medicating had gotten out of control, but what I didn't realize was that she had a disease that was spreading and that it had multiplied and crossed the blood-brain barrier, which caused a reaction in her that was similar to the way syphilis can cause psychosis. I tried to convince her to go to a rehabilitation hospital, but, as could be expected, she wouldn't hear it. I thought she might have been on psychedelic drugs, but she insisted she wasn't. So I decided that out of love for my daughter, I was going to have to use force. Two of my security guards helped me put her into a car to bring her to the emergency room and eventually Silver Hill Hospital, a psychiatric and addiction rehabilitation facility in Connecticut.

During that dark time, I knew Ally was very angry at me. I can still see the look on my daughter's face when she thought I'd turned on her when she needed me most. One of the reasons I was so distraught and acted so dramatically is that I was quite aware of the teenage suicide rate and that thought haunted me; it was always in the back of my mind. If something like that were to happen I could never forgive myself.

So, I thought I had to save her life, and I was going to do whatever I had to do, and however I had to do it. Believe me, this was traumatic for all of us. I never gave up hope, however, that she would eventually see that love was my primary motivation.

As a father, there is nothing more devastating than seeing your child suffer and go through intense pain, except, perhaps, seeing her suffer and not knowing why. Silver Hill Hospital turned out to be a godsend. It was there that Ally would meet Dr. Ellyn Shander, who would properly diagnose her for the first time. Thank God for Dr. Shander.

Finding out what had been causing Ally's physical and emotional pain was a relief, but it proved to be only the beginning of a journey that never seems to end. No matter how dormant her disease seemed, we lived in constant fear and worry that at any minute it would raise its ugly head. And it did, over and over again.

This disease is an uncontrolled, widespread epidemic, and what makes things even more difficult is that a lot of people don't know they have it. They're living with all sorts of ailments and don't realize what's causing them—and the longer it sits in your body, the worse it gets. With Lyme, there is no real, certain cure.

When I now see Ally holding my healthy, happy granddaughter, Harley, I know that she feels the same way I did when I held her for the first time in a cab. I'm incredibly proud of my daughter, for all she has withstood, all she has accomplished, and for the loving, giving person she is.

This book is testament of her giving nature, a gift of hope for those who suffer from Lyme disease and to anyone who has ever overcome a challenge, whatever it may be.

—Tommy Hilfiger

preface

I don't remember when I was bit. It might have been in the summer of 1991 or '92. My mother does, but she's not sure where it happened. It could've been on Nantucket, or in Bridgehampton, New York, or even in our yard in Greenwich, Connecticut, she thinks. Though she doesn't remember where it happened, she does remember finding the minuscule black creature with eight legs on my tummy, right next to my funny-shaped birthmark. Mom remembers too that she did exactly what the pediatricians were telling mothers to do: She pulled the tick off of me with sterile tweezers, put it in a test tube, and brought it to have it tested. The tests came back "inconclusive" but leaned more toward the negative side of the spectrum. My parents were dissatisfied with "inconclusive" results and decided to seek out a specialist. Unfortunately they were not given any hope or a list of symptoms to look out for. My mother is still very perplexed by the way the specialist handled the situation.

Studies now find that some 50 percent of commonly used Lyme testing misses positive Lyme cases.

Fifty percent!

It's fitting somehow, though, that neither my mom nor I remember where the bite occurred and that doctors missed the correct diagnosis. Lyme disease is as sneaky as it is nasty: About half of the people infected by Lyme are like me: They can't tell you when they were bitten. A very small percentage of people who have been bitten by a tick recall a bull's-eye rash, which for years has been the medical community's common indicator that a person has Lyme. In fact, before it even bites you, the tick releases a combination of chemicals that act like an anesthetic, so most times you don't even know the little bloodsucker is burrowing into you. This is not a mosquito bite, people. Ticks can attach themselves to you for days because it takes that long for the spirochete bacteria to make its way into your bloodstream. Then it can take up to three weeks before you feel that anything's wrong, and even then, most people think they just have the flu.

What happens next is where it gets really devious. Fact: After they have been bit, most people wait two and a half years to receive a proper diagnosis. Lyme can mimic any number of illnesses. Believe me, I know. During my Lyme life, doctors would diagnose me with everything from mono to multiple sclerosis and dozens of other diseases in between, and in spite of a mountain of symptomatic evidence that supported the fact that I had Lyme, doctors would refuse to diagnose me with it because of the ambiguous results of the tests I was given.

They call Lyme "the invisible disease" or "the great imitator," as if it's some kind of world-renowned stage actor. I can think of a couple of other names for it that aren't quite as complimentary. From the age of seven or eight, I experienced Lyme-created nightmares of sickness, hospitalizations, disappointments, and depression. Yet, in a kind of perverse way, it has also been a gift. Because of it, I found an inner strength that I couldn't have imagined. It's a good thing, too. Because I would need every ounce of that strength just to survive.

I'm not some kind of singular hero, though. In fact, my Lyme story is, literally, one in a million. According to the U.S. Centers for Disease Control and Prevention (CDC) there are thirty-four new cases of Lyme every hour, and all of us are battling not only our illness but a backlash of medical misconception, misinformation, and misdiagnosis. There are doctors right now, ones with diplomas from impressive medical schools hanging on their walls, who deny the reaches of this horrible disease. There are loving and caring family members who refuse to believe that their son, daughter, brother, or sister is really suffering from Lyme's effects. There are far, far too many who are never diagnosed and who couldn't afford the treatment if they were.

No, my story is not unusual, but I believe it needs to be told if only to give others a voice for theirs.

Before I start telling it, though, I need to warn you of something: Lyme disease is a thief, and it not only steals your ability to live a normal life, it also swipes your memories just as soon as you turn your back. It's like a junkie acquaintance. A lot of my childhood, and even my teenage and young adult years, are lost in the fog of Lyme. In high school, I often walked the streets of New York City with a video camera so I could capture the moments I was afraid I'd forget. In my twenties I hung a Polaroid camera around my neck for the same reason. I literally covered the walls in my rooms with photos I took from that camera.

For the sake of this book, I researched much of my own life by asking family and friends to fill the holes in my memory. I also kept journals for periods of my teen and young adult years, and luckily those diaries survived my many moves. Reading them again did bring back many details that I'd forgotten. Some of the recollections I'll recount in the pages ahead came shrieking back to me like a strip of film pulled from a projector—a flash of video consciousness, if you will. Those recollections I'll play back for you just as I remember them.

When pieced together, hopefully these memories will start to make sense of a life of which I had little understanding for a very long time.

part one

one

A BITE OF CRAZY

> ➤ *"Lyme disease is a multisystemic illness that can affect the central nervous system (CNS), causing neurologic and psychiatric symptoms."*[1]
> —National Institutes of Health

In late December 2003, just a few weeks after the last airing of a reality television show I'd starred in, I opened my eyes in a strange, dark room with cinder-block walls, and in a bed made for an elf. Perhaps most disturbing was the fact that my orange and red Adidas sneakers were missing their laces. I looked down at the inside of my arm, which was itching, and saw a piece of gauze being held in place by a Band-Aid.

Am I in a hospital? Did I try to hurt myself? Am I in a mental institution? Am I in jail? I could barely think because my head was pounding so badly.

I managed to pull myself up but my head started to spin, so I lay back down and tears began to roll down my face. *Where am I?* I felt alone, scared, and I could not remember a thing. I recognized the familiar confusion, loneliness, fear, and head pain. I needed to wake myself up from this dream, this nightmare. The nightmare I had been living my whole life.

I walked into the hall, a brightly lighted, carpeted corridor. There was a window with bars, and outside these windows I saw snow-covered trees. The landscape looked like somewhere on the East Coast. *Maybe I am close to home.* I wanted to go home and just be held and comforted in my mother's arms. As I turned around I wiped away tears and suddenly a large redheaded man was guiding me toward the end of the hallway to a chair.

"Where am I? Where are you taking me?" I asked the man.

"We have to take your blood pressure and temperature," he said.

"Why? Where am I? What's happening?"

"You are at Silver Hill Hospital in the Acute Care Unit."

My heart dropped to the pit of my stomach and I was in complete shock. *I have been totally misunderstood,* I thought, *and thrown into a nuthouse without my consent.*

My dad did this, I thought. A father should walk you down the aisle, not walk you down a locked corridor. *How could my dad do this to me?* I had always trusted him more than anyone. He had always been the one I called when I felt lost, sad, and uncertain. So the question of what had happened to me became, what had happened to me and my dad?

Our relationship was never like this when I was younger.

When I was four years old, every Saturday morning my dad would put me on the back of his bicycle to go for a ride through the back roads of our pretty town. He would stop near the water, and we would sit and stare in awe and amusement. After the bike ride, he would take me to the mall for curly fries and an A&W root beer. Saturdays were my absolute favorite because I was with my favorite person in the world. My father understood me like no one else, stood up for me, believed in me, and encouraged me. I always felt safe when I was in his presence. Always.

Not, however, today.

At night, after my mom sang me her homemade lullabies, put me in my foot pajamas, and tucked me in, I would wait for my father to come home from work in the city and give me a kiss good night. He would rush to get home before I fell asleep and I fought to keep my eyes open until he was home.

Now at eighteen years old, I was curled up at the bottom of a bed waiting again for my knight in shining armor to come and save me. Save me from the nuthouse. It was my knight, however, who drugged me and locked me up in this place. I tried to remember if Christmas had passed but couldn't. Everything was a blur.

The last thing I remembered was going to a church to beg a priest to bestow sleep upon me. Sleep was a battle, and I rarely won. I wanted so desperately to be able to put my head on a pillow and easily drift into a dream world, but instead I was living in a state of wide-awake paranoia. The last episode of the TV show that had ruined my life had just aired, and I couldn't walk into a gas station without being recognized. I thought someone was out to get me and that stalkers waited around every corner to attack me. I felt alone, frightened, and convinced that some dark force was keeping me from sleeping or having any sort of appetite, not to mention giving me the persistent nausea and joint pain I was unable to ignore.

I remembered walking into a little stone church in the center of Bedford Village, New York, on Christmas Eve carrying every spiritual book my mother had ever given me, a few pine tree branches that I smelled to relieve nausea, and a head of grungy hair that featured two dreadlocks. I had become that person, that homeless woman you see on the sidewalk passing out pamphlets on Forty-Ninth Street, talking to herself.

After the mass I decided to go up to random people I thought might need spiritual saving and hand them a copy of *The Power of Now* or Mother Teresa's *In My Own Words*. These books had given me hope and it was my assumption that they might help other lost souls in the crowded Christmas Eve mass.

As I lay on that little elf-sized bed, I remembered, too, a few weeks before Christmas, when I was on my father's bathroom floor crying in pain, and he choked up and asked me, "What can I do? How can I help? Anything, I will do anything to help you and make you feel better."

"Pot," I said to him. "Get me some pot. It's the only thing that will help me."

The excruciating joint pain and flulike symptoms had been part of my life since I was a little girl. My parents and doctors dismissed my complaints about my knees feeling achy and hot. I was told they were growing pains. They treated the constant bouts of strep throat with bubble-gum-flavored antibiotic and never looked into my health in any comprehensive manner.

As the years went on, I felt as though my brain was not working as well as the other kids' in my class. When I got tested, they told me I had attention deficit disorder, ADD. When I stopped being able to read, they said I had a learning disability and sent me to a specialist. When I couldn't remember the information I had studied for four hours the night before a test, they told me to study harder. When I couldn't wake up for school or keep my eyes open during class, they told me I needed to go to bed earlier and exercise more. When I told them I had pounding headaches several days a week, they told me to drink more water or "pop a couple of Advils," even when the headache was so strong I couldn't lift my head from my desk. When I was in agony from severe hip pain and random joint pain, they said, "It's probably rheumatoid arthritis. Or maybe it's multiple sclerosis. Or it sounds like fibromyalgia. Or it could be . . ."

Who is "they," you ask? My parents, teachers, doctors, and the people in between.

Speaking of doctors, the one at Silver Hill was a piece of work. Let's just say he took himself really seriously. When he walked into my room, the first thing I noticed was that his suit was a little too nice, and his shirt was a little too pressed, and his tie matched his socks. He arrived with an arrogant disposition, which made me feel immediately judged and belittled.

My cousin had come to visit me the day before, and she'd brought me a crazy orange and fuchsia hat with those wild pom-poms with long tassels sticking out all over the top. Ha! Little did this stern, buttoned-up doctor know he would be forced into wearing this hat atop his ensemble or else I would not speak or even look at him.

I just needed this guy to drop back down to earth. Or slightly above earth in my case, in another realm of playfulness and spirituality (or just plain old psychosis) that was my defense against the pain I was in on a daily basis. I wasn't being silly because I was incapable of being serious. I was being silly because I was terrified. I was not sure what he was treating me for or what he thought was wrong with me.

In my room at Silver Hill, I had my necessities: one tiny wooden Ganesh, a Hindu deity with an elephant head who removes obstacles, a book on infinity with the ∞ symbol on the front, a deck of cards, a journal, a sketch pad, Chapstick, and a pack of Marlboro Lights. I didn't care about showering or clothing or any of that superficial madness; yes, showering is superficial when you're on lockdown. I was so tired of image and material things.

On one of the first days at the hospital I had a flashback of a day that had certainly led up to my being in this place. I had been angry at my parents for not listening to me when I said I didn't feel well; they seemed too preoccupied with work and money and making the house look good. I exploded and raged and screamed and cried, and I broke one of my mother's favorite plates. (You can't have a nervous breakdown without breaking expensive plates. Ask Edward Albee.)

All eighty-five pounds of me was coming undone. For days I hadn't been able to eat, shower, or sleep. I was convinced that bugs were crawling in my body. I could feel them eating at my organs, my stomach, and especially my brain. I wasn't me anymore. I was a weakly projected image of myself on a wall, crying out for someone to help me and figure out what was wrong.

Well, my dad did just that, but never in my wildest dreams did I think he would help me in the dramatic way he chose.

Staring into the eyes of this doctor in his shiny suit made me feel crazier and more emotional. The colorful snowboarding hat only went so far. I realized no one was going to help me get out of here, no one was going to listen to what was really going on. No one was going to believe that I used the marijuana found in my blood to help me eat something without feeling as if I was going to vomit, and to help me sleep. No one was going to understand that this wasn't the place that I needed to be.

Except the one person who would. I'd had a vague dream of someone who had the power or authority to get me out of here and find the missing piece to my health puzzle. This person was the answer and the key to my ultimate freedom from it all.

I had no idea I had to go through weeks of hellish existence in order to figure out who this phantom person was.

two

FASHION FAIRY TALE

*"Lyme is also destroying families, and the really sad thing is, a
serious illness is when people need their families the most."*[2]
—JORDON FISHER SMITH, NARRATOR AND SUBJECT
OF THE AWARD-WINNING LYME DISEASE
DOCUMENTARY *UNDER OUR SKIN*

So how did I actually end up in a nuthouse? Well, to get the full
answer you have to go back to the beginning. All life stories start
with a set of parents. My dad grew up about as small-town as you
can get. Two hundred and thirty miles northwest of Manhattan,
Elmira, New York, has a population of thirty thousand on a good
day—of which there aren't many since a lot of the factories closed in
the 1970s. My dad lived in a small house on 606 West Clinton Street
with eight brothers and sisters. He was the second child, the oldest
boy, and he didn't have it easy. His father would get drunk and beat
my dad with a belt. My grandfather's name was Richard but they
called him Hippo. Family lore has it that Hippo got the name when
he was playing high school football. Small in stature, my grandfather had a ferocity that belied his size.

My grandfather worked in a jewelry store, where he fixed and made watches and jewelry, and Virginia, my grandmother, whom we called Nonnie, was a nurse. Nonnie was a saint, a beloved figure in my family.

From the moment he was able, my dad worked as hard as he could. He mowed lawns, shoveled snow, delivered newspapers, and worked nights in a gas station for $1.25 an hour, anything to put some cash in his pocket, or, as he says, "to buy a pair of sneakers." He also helped his family financially.

What defined my dad best back then was probably rock and roll. He grew up in the sixties and loved listening to the Who; the Rolling Stones; Crosby, Stills, Nash & Young; Eric Clapton; and all the other now-"classic" rock bands.

My father's career in fashion began in the summer of 1969 when he was a senior in high school. He and a couple of friends went to Cape Cod, where Dad got a job in what he now calls a "boutique" but what was essentially a head shop that sold incense, T-shirts, and band posters. He loved his experience on the Cape. When he returned to Elmira he jumped into his Volkswagen Beetle and drove to New York City with $150 he'd saved from working nights in the gas station and bought twenty pairs of bell-bottom jeans on St. Marks Place, in Greenwich Village. Back home, he rented a basement space, painted it black, played the Who on his stereo, and sold the jeans along with fringed vests and other items. The hippie bell-bottom and fringed-vest attire hadn't yet reached Elmira. He called his store People's Place and it was enough of a hit that he soon opened another one in nearby Ithaca on the Cornell University campus.

It was in the store in Ithaca that Susie Cirona, my mom, worked. She was fifteen when she started. The Cornell campus also played a role in her father's life. My grandfather, Jim Cirona, graduated from the university. The design gene on my mother's side of the family came from her grandfather, who emigrated from Sicily and became a tailor in Little Italy in New York City. Mom remembers the coats he made for her and her siblings to wear to Mass on Sundays.

My mother's Greek grandmother lived in the house in which my mom grew up. As my mother remembers, her nana was a soft, humble, sweet, and loving woman. She had supper with my mom and her four siblings every evening. I think my mother adopted her nana's compassionate, soft, and loving ways. Mom's affinity for nature began in her early childhood. She would collect caterpillars and put them in her baby doll carriage, and she cut fresh lilacs and put them in her room. Later she would spend the majority of her time in the woods and on her bicycle. Mom was shy as a child, at least with people she didn't know well. She was devoted to her father, a kind, loving, and patient man. Her parents took her out of Catholic school and put her in the public school in the hope of opening her up. At home, however, she kept her brother and three sisters laughing. Once in the middle of a summer heat wave, she walked around the un-air-conditioned house dressed in layers and layers of winter clothing, cracking everyone up. Mom sewed many of her own clothes and, in fact, was accepted into the Fashion Institute of Technology in Manhattan because of a dress she made herself.

My mother tells me that she began to work for my dad after his partner, who ran the Ithaca store, fired her. She hitchhiked all the way to Elmira, about forty miles, to complain and my dad gave her a job at his store. They started dating soon after.

In 1979, my parents moved together to New York City to follow a dream of a life in fashion. Not too long before, People's Place had gone bankrupt, an event my father calls "his master's degree in business," so my parents started with practically nothing. Mom and Dad didn't have a lot of money then. They first lived in a tiny apartment on Thirty-First Street, on the same floor as a gay couple, which they thought was very hip and cutting edge back then, and a mysterious man and woman who seemed to never leave the apartment. At the time, my parents would scrounge up the money to travel to India to make their clothing designs. They returned from one trip to find the door of their mysterious neighbors' apartment riddled with bullet holes. The FBI had raided the place. Apparently, the man was on their Most Wanted List.

Despite their rough beginnings, neither of them lost faith. My mom has always had a very intense intuition and foresight, which fit perfectly with dad's innate ability to sniff out liars and inauthentic people, a talent that, over the years, I've been able to hone myself. But he too had a clear vision of his future. My mom says she confronted him one day, years before his career began to take off, by asking what he wanted from his life. "I want to be as famous as Calvin Klein, Perry Ellis, and Ralph Lauren," he said.

Soon after, they moved to Ninth Street between First Avenue and Avenue A. It wasn't much of an improvement. Though today it is a center of hipsters and college kids, the East Village back then was heroin central and about as dangerous a neighborhood you could find in Manhattan. My dad says he and my mom were in their punk phase. They hung out in places like CBGB's, the birthplace of New York City's punk rock music. They met Andy Warhol, and managed to dodge the drug deals and gunfire that were common occurrences in their neighborhood. They also went to Studio 54 and got into the famously selective club because of the way they dressed: Mom in a leopard coat and white sunglasses, and dad in a leather bomber jacket.

Both of my parents had a number of stops and starts in their careers before anything clicked. Jordache jeans fired them both after a month, as did Bon Jour jeans. Like my dad, my mom has great taste and a lot of talent and when they both started designing their own collections, it looked as though my mom was going to be the more successful one.

In New York, my dad had started a clothing line then called 20th Century Survival, which was doing pretty well. It sold at Macy's, Saks Fifth Avenue, and Neiman Marcus. At the same time, my mother started her own women's sportswear collection called O Tokyo and it was a massive hit, much bigger than my father's collection. O Tokyo was in some of the city's best stores, such as Henri Bendel and Bloomingdale's.

As it happened, my father and mother both had shows during the same Fashion Week and my mother's collection received far more publicity. She was the It Girl, the new, exciting designer of her day. The guys involved in my father's company said to him, "You might want to ask the wife to step aside a little. She's getting all the attention."

My father would never do that. Instead he came up with a better idea: He got my mom pregnant with me. When my mom went to Tokyo to work on her collection for the last time she was several months into her pregnancy.

I was born at New York University Medical Center on February 26, 1985. My dad remembers the event so clearly he can tell you what he was wearing: khaki pants, a baggy varsity cardigan sweater, blue and white button-down oxford shirt, and white K-Swiss sneakers.

My mother's memories of my coming into the world were far less superficial. Her hair had morphed into a disastrous mess of knots and her eyes were bloodshot from all of the screaming and swearing.

Apparently the doctor had a golf game to get to and induced labor with so much Pitocin that the epidural didn't even work. Explains why she waited five years to get pregnant again. Who could blame the poor woman?

After I was born, my parents moved to Sixty-Eighth Street between Central Park West and Columbus Avenue. My dad tells me that the night they took me home I slept in a bassinette at the foot of their bed. He kept getting up and putting his finger under my nose to see if I was breathing because I slept so quietly. Years later, when our relationship wasn't nearly as sedate, to say the least, I'm sure my dad yearned for that innocent time.

My dad always said I was his lucky charm. In 1985, the year I was born, he opened the Tommy Hilfiger store on Columbus Avenue, was asked to design the Coca-Cola clothing line, and launched his first Tommy Hilfiger collection. In case you ever wondered why my father uses the number 85 on his clothing, now you know.

In one sense, I came along at just the right moment, when the stars of the fashion universe were aligned in our favor. I was born into a fairy tale waiting to happen. It was a blessed beginning. If that little bug with eight legs hadn't crawled its way into our lives, it might have been a life too good to be true.

three
"OFF TO SEE THE WIZARD..."

"In children and adolescents, Lyme disease can also mimic specific or pervasive developmental delays, attention-deficit disorder (inattentive subtype), oppositional defiant disorder, mood disorders, obsessive-compulsive disorder (OCD), anorexia, Tourette's syndrome, and pseudopsychotic disorders."
—RICHARD I. HOROWITZ, M.D.

Maybe the worst part of any Lyme story is the *What if?* of it. Children ages three to fourteen are at the greatest risk of contracting the disease, and if they contract it, they are haunted and hunted by it for the rest of their lives. There was a time, however, when I couldn't imagine my life being anything but pretty wonderful.

When I was ten months old we moved from Manhattan to Greenwich, Connecticut. Our house on Round Hill Road was a colonial in the traditional sense except for the pink carpeting that covered the floors. I remember waking up early and curling up into a ball on that carpet in front of my parents' bedroom door. I'd lie there, sucking my thumb, until they awoke.

Here are some other fragmented memories I have from that time:

When I was very young I had a nanny named Maggie, then a Polish nanny named Alice, who would make fairy crowns for me out of daisies and dandelions from the yard.

My parents called me Bunny Bun.

There was a little white wooden playhouse in the yard. It had green shutters, a shingled roof, and a little porch (we still have it!). I would always play house in it, pretending to cook and clean in the four-foot by six-foot building. We still have pictures of me sweeping the front porch. The song "In My Own Little Corner" from Rodgers and Hammerstein's *Cinderella* always reminds me of being in that house.

I began ballet classes and my teacher's name was Mrs. Foote! I loved my ballet costume, a tutu, and I always wanted wear it. My mother says that in those days I "bounced with sunshine."

My bedroom had a white wrought-iron bed and a white wicker rocking chair. A seamstress named Rachel made custom clothing for my mother. Rachel would come to the house to go over fabrics and colors with my mother every season. Rachel gave me a stuffed dog I named Mutsy. After I was bitten by the tick, I would hold Mutsy between my knees to ease the pain in my joints so I could sleep.

I'd spend hours coloring in a playroom off my bedroom. There my dad and I played a game we called Store. I had a vegetable stand with plastic veggies, and we would be the managers. And he would say, "Alexandria, Mrs. Jones just called and she would like three tomatoes and two cucumbers." I put the plastic vegetables in a little bag. Then he'd say, "Mr. Roberts just called and he would like a pepper along with his oranges." Dad would play with me for hours.

We had a huge front yard and used to jump in the leaves together, play hide-and-seek in the woods, and ice-skate on the pond behind the house. Dad called me his Princess Alexandria. Clichéd, I know, but we really had such a special connection. It was as if we were soul mates in a past life meeting again in this one. Our closeness was powerful and very tangible.

I was close with my mom, too, when I was little. Together we made meatballs and watched reruns of *Gilligan's Island*, *I Love Lucy*, and *I Dream of Jeannie*. I watched *Cinderella* and *The Wizard of Oz* until the VHS tapes were creased and faded. I remember the baths we took together in her big bathtub. She would hold me after the bath and rock and sing to me. It was my favorite time with her.

I didn't, however, like the way mom dressed me! She'd have me wear smock dresses with Peter Pan collars, wool cardigans, and blazers. They might have been nice clothes, but to me they were just itchy and confining. The shoes I wore were so tight you had to button them with a special contraption that was like a hanger. I didn't like them at all.

I had one pair of shoes, though, that I wouldn't take off my feet. They were little beaded, red velvet slippers that my father brought back from a business trip to Hong Kong. I think I even slept with them on, and I still have them. I wore the red slippers with blue cotton pants that my mother and I called "summer pants." I wanted to wear the summer pants all the time and did until one day, when I was sitting on the ground and fire ants ate away at them. I was so upset. Of all my outfits, my least favorite was a turtleneck and corduroy overalls, which my mother dressed me in every time I was sick. To this day, if I put on a turtleneck or overalls I get this feeling I'm going to throw up or have explosive diarrhea.

Around that time, my mom opened a children's clothing store called Beauchamp Place, in Greenwich, with a woman named Nancy Seaman. My mom was always working at the store, which was becoming successful, and my dad had started making a name in business. Still, it wasn't as though the money was rolling in. In fact, my parents now admit they were living far beyond their means. There was one time they had to borrow oil from Mr. Strain's gas station on Round Hill Road to heat the house. By this time I guess we were trying to keep up with the Greenwich Joneses.

My dad stayed close to his siblings and mother and they were always visiting. There were two attic bedrooms in the house on Round Hill Road. My aunt Ginny slept in one while she was at the Fashion Institute of Technology (the same school my mom attended for a semester) and my uncle Billy lived in the attic for a short while when he was in a band with my uncle Andy. I remember my mother dressing my uncles in Civil War costumes for one photo shoot.

It was Uncle Andy who in 1994 was responsible for my father's biggest break in his career. Andy lived in East Harlem and would listen to music in the clubs. It was there he met a rapper named Snoop Dogg. Andy offered Snoop some Tommy Hilfiger gear to wear for an appearance on *Saturday Night Live*. The night of the show, the rapper wore one of my father's rugby shirts with Tommy emblazoned across the front. After that everything changed for all of us, but I didn't realize it until many years later. My parents tried very hard to keep me sheltered from the attention my father began to receive. In school, kids began to say things like, "Oh, you must be really rich," or "Your parents must be millionaires," but as a child, I was truly naïve about it all.

Growing up, I loved all of my father's family and continue to do so. Kathy, Susie, Betsy, Bobby, Billy, Dee Dee, Andy, and Ginny were my dad's siblings, and they all played wonderful roles in my life. They were and still are great influencers. But my uncle Billy held a special place in my heart and I held a special place in his heart, too.

He wrote a song for me and called it "Alexandria." I still know all the words, but when I was little I'd be embarrassed when he'd sing it at a family gathering. Now when I think of that song and start to hum it, I cry.

My parents loved to look at houses and go antiquing and they took me along. I only wanted to go in the car to visit Aunt Betsy and her sons, Mike and Joe, and Nonnie, of course. To me, the antiquing trips were the most boring things in the world. When we turned onto the Merritt Parkway I'd know where we were going and cry out from the backseat: "Oh no! Not the highway!"

My dad drove an old sedan, navy blue, with caramel tan interior. I'd lie down on the backseat and count the little indentations in the leather. Most of the time I'd just fall asleep and when they returned home my parents would leave me napping in the car, parked in front of our house. I remember waking up horrified that I was alone. To this day it still freaks me out when I wake up alone from a nap.

But in the car they'd play Joni Mitchell; Carole King; and Crosby, Stills, Nash & Young on the tape deck. It was on those trips that my love of rock and roll was born. I can still remember my favorite song at the time, "Our House," by Crosby, Stills, Nash & Young.

When I was little, we'd also go on vacation to Nantucket. We'd drive onto the beach, open the back of our old Range Rover and play the Rolling Stones and go fishing. My parents rented houses in Bridgehampton and Water Mill, New York, during a few summers. My only memory of vacationing on Long Island is behind the house we rented in Bridgehampton. There was a little hill of grass, with baby pines that reached my waist. My parents were trying to get me to stop sucking my thumb. I had a bar across my mouth the orthodontist had prescribed. But I'd go up to my little fortress among the pine trees and suck my thumb to my heart's content. I did it so much I put a dent in the bar.

My favorite vacation back then was visiting Nonnie and Betsy up in Elmira. The home on West Clinton Street was a small white wood Victorian with a little tower on the corner, which I called the castle tower. I used to go up into Nonnie's attic and play dress-up with her old clothes. The backyard was about two hundred square feet and was filled with my grandpa Hippo's rosebushes. Grandpa Hippo had a charming side and Nonnie loved him dearly. During the winter, Hippo brought the rosebushes inside, where they'd lie dormant in the laundry room in their basement. On the first Valentine's Day after Hippo died in December 1990, when I was about five, Nonnie went down to the basement to flip the laundry. When she turned around to go upstairs she noticed a large red rose had bloomed on one of the bushes. In the dead of winter!

Nonnie made us tomato sandwiches with salt and pepper and she always served Entenmann's powdered donuts and Folger's coffee. She sent us Gap pajamas every Christmas. Her sister, my father's aunt Annie, lived nearby. Her house was surrounded by pussy willows that I loved to touch. Annie was very strict—she was the one who taught my father manners, which are impeccable. She'd say to him, "If you're truly a well-mannered boy you'll get far in life." Her husband, Bill, had a buzz cut, and he was scared shitless of Annie.

Aunt Annie could scare the living shit out of me, too. She'd say things like, "If you don't be quiet I'm going to take a round out of your shorts!" She looked after us one summer when my parents went to Europe, and all I remember from that time is crying a lot. Annie had a stern face, curly reddish brown hair, dark maroon lipstick, and drawn-on eyebrows, which she taught me how to draw. She also taught me the trick of taking a bit of lipstick and putting it on the apples of your cheeks to give them a little color, and how to pull stockings up over your knees without getting snags in them.

Like all the Hilfigers, Annie worked hard. She was a typist and secretary, and like the rest of my father's family she also had a pretty good sense of humor. In the 1950s, Nonnie and Hippo had bridge night, with a foldout table, endless amounts of cigarettes, and cheap hors d'oeuvres. One night, one of the husbands from the other couples who joined the game put his hand on Aunt Annie's knee under the table. She looked him right in the eye and said, "What's the matter? Not happy at home?"

On vacations to Elmira, I got to see my aunt Betsy and my cousins Mike and Joe, who were a few years older than I was. I remember being at the Piggly Wiggly market and climbing into the basket of a cart. Joe crawled into the space underneath the basket and Mike pushed us so fast down the aisle I peed on Joe's head. I was laughing so hard I just peed. Mike had to take some paper towels off the shelf to dry his brother's hair.

The childhood vacation that had the biggest impact on my life, however, was one I don't really remember—I was just nine months old. The destination was a small private island in the Caribbean called Mustique. By 1985, my parents had started making some money and vacationed in St. Barths, but when it became too crowded with New Yorkers, they searched for a more private and quiet Caribbean island to go to. They discovered Mustique and fell in love with it. They ended up buying a home called Pamplemousse (French for grapefruit) on L'Ansecoy Bay, which is on the north side of the island. The house was next to Mick Jagger's and Bryan Adams's homes, as it happened.

I also fell in love with Mustique, and the island became an integral part of my life and life's story. There's magic in Mustique, maybe because it has a huge crystal vein running through it. Or maybe because it's just that kind of special place. I consider the people who live, work, and own homes on Mustique as my extended family. My soul lives there with the crystals that grow wild out of the earth, the grape-seed leaves that flourish in the dunes of the beaches, and the bright yellow sea fans that sway to and fro in the clear Caribbean Sea. I was always a bit melancholy when we'd leave the island.

In fact, when I was sixteen years old I decided not to leave.

We were scheduled for a one o'clock hopper plane to leave the island with my grandfather and mom. Along with my friends Garrett and Danielle and my two younger siblings, I planned the scheme the night before. We'd hide on a little beach that I knew my mother and grandfather didn't know about. The next day, we were there for hours giggling and playing in the sand and sea, without a care in the world, so proud of our cheeky adventure. My younger siblings were tempted to chicken out but they didn't need too much convincing to stay that day.

Back on our little hideaway beach, we were so pleased when the clock passed the one o'clock point. We did it! All of a sudden an old Land Cruiser pulled up. The driver was Mick Jagger's then-companion Jerry Hall, who had been sent out with others to search for us. We grew up with the Jagger children, and our families have remained very close over the years. She found the five of us huddled up in the sand, trying to become invisible. She told us that my mom and grandfather were not happy. Oops! Then she drove us to the airport. We arrived there sandy, wet, and in our swimwear, all with our tails between our legs. They made us get on the plane that way. It was a long trip back, to say the least.

* * *

My brother Richard's birth on March 28, 1990, was a huge event for me (I'm sure it was for him, too). I had dolls as a child and when my mother was pregnant I practiced holding them like babies so I'd be ready when my brother arrived. When he did, I kept asking to hold him and I'd sit with him in the back of the car when he was taking his naps.

I am the eldest of four. My brother Richard is five years younger, Elizabeth is eight years younger, and Kathleen is eleven years younger than I am. I thought they were my babies, and they treated me like their mom. I developed strong maternal instincts for all of my siblings.

In 1990, when Richard was a couple of months old, we moved back to Manhattan. I was five. We lived in a townhouse on East Eightieth Street. I remember acting grown-up in taxis with my parents. I'd insist on telling the cabdriver our address and would emulate my mother: "One, two, three East Eightieth Street between Park and Lex," I'd say. "That's eight zero." I also emulated the way my mother spells our last name to people over the telephone: "H-I-L-F as in Frank-I-G-E-R." I still do it to this day.

On Eightieth Street, Whoopi Goldberg was our neighbor. I don't mean to name-drop, but you have to allow me a totally random Whoopi Goldberg story. A few years ago, I went to a show during Fashion Week and Whoopi was sitting a few seats away from me. I got the courage to introduce myself and say that I thought she was just awesome, that I admired her career, and so on. Whoopi then asked if I was Tommy's daughter. I told her I was. "Oh my God," she said. "Your father's in my will."

Naturally I was interested as to why my father would be in Whoopi Goldberg's will. Here's the story she told me: Years before, she'd gone to the Sotheby's auction for the Duke and Duchess of

Windsor's furniture. My parents were also there and they ended up bidding against Whoopi for a chaise longue. My father bought a large lot, which included the chaise, but somehow the chair was accidentally delivered to Whoopi's house. "I put your dad in my will," she told me, "because when I die I want the chaise longue to go back to him."

The townhouse we lived in had five floors. I remember zooming down the flights of stairs in a sleeping bag like a toboggan. We had rabbits, and we kept them in the downstairs kitchen when it was too cold for them outside.

The top floor was a sunroom, with big glass windows facing the street and a glass-domed roof. I remember it had blue carpeting and tons of toys. There were two huge mirrors in the bathroom and when you looked in one mirror you could see yourself in the other, and that reflection would reflect in the other and on and on forever, it seemed. It was in that bathroom that I became aware of my physical self and was surprised by it. When I looked at all my reflections it was as if my brain opened up, expanded beyond reality. I felt as if I was outside myself with a thousand me's. Today they might call it "meta reality." I remember thinking I didn't know who all those reflections were looking back at me. It really tripped me out. It was as though I was surprised I owned the human body I wore. I'd had to leave the bathroom and go play with something that would get me out of my head and back to the real world.

The Ally I remember from the townhouse on East Eightieth was a little girl whose world was a stage, and she was the starlet ferociously taking charge of the role she felt she deserved. My father was like the producer of the play with his sweet, gentle, yet strong presence that made me feel as though everything was going to be okay. My mother, on the other hand, was the fed-up writer or director who just wanted to get on with the show. To this day, she feels that I have the temperament of the great actresses; she calls me a blend of Elizabeth Taylor, Bette Davis, Meryl Streep, and possibly Katharine Hepburn. I'm not sure if I can take that as a compliment 100 percent of the time, but I'll take it when it is!

My parents took me to see my first therapist when I was six. Mom and Dad wanted to do everything they could to offer as much support as possible as my father grew more successful. The office was on Christopher Street in Greenwich Village, and the lady therapist would let me put on her lipstick and play checkers with me. There was big dollhouse in the office, and I'd always put all the dolls in the same room instead of spreading them throughout the house. I wanted the family to be cozy together in one room.

I was also enrolled in kindergarten at the Hewitt School at the time, though that experience is mostly lost. I do remember my kindergarten teachers' names were Ms. Pearl and Ms. Nothumb, which strikes me now as hysterically funny since I was an addicted thumb sucker as a child. I remember too that we wore navy and green plaid jumpers and did gymnastics.

I began my Catholic school career in first grade at the Convent of the Sacred Heart, on East Ninety-First Street. I wore a gray jumper with a red and white gingham pinafore. I was infatuated with the nuns and their getups. I asked one, an older nun, to take off the headpiece of her habit so I could see what was underneath. She did, and her hair was clipped up in all these multicolored plastic bow clips! Every morning we had to get in line and shake the headmistress's hand and curtsey, right foot behind the left. I remember practicing my curtsey.

It was while we were still living on East Eightieth that my life began to change. Random outbursts of rage occurred out of nowhere. I realize now that it was not long before that I had been bitten by that infected tick. I learned later that emotional outbursts are a common side effect from acute Lyme disease. Back then, however, Lyme wasn't even a suspect.

four

SCARED HEART AND
GROWING PAINS

*"The usual laboratory tests alone are not totally reliable to confirm
or refute the diagnosis of Lyme disease. When we combine the
current laboratory tests with a very thorough history, physical, and
mental status exam, the accuracy of diagnosis is greatly increased."*
—ROBERT BRANSFIELD, M.D.

In the late 1970s scientists began wondering why a group of young
hikers near the town of Lyme, Connecticut, had started develop-
ing mysterious symptoms like swollen joints, unusual rashes, and
fevers. In fact, however, the illness had been brought to the attention of the medical community years earlier. A woman named
Polly Murray, along with her whole family, had suffered from Lyme
symptoms as far back as the 1960s. Her doctors diagnosed juvenile
rheumatoid arthritis and some type of an obscure trauma, and they
refused to believe it was anything else. The medical community literally brushed her aside.[3]

Dissatisfied with their conclusions, she didn't give up seeking
a true diagnosis. In the 1970s, a doctor named Allen Steele figured
out that a tick, which fed on deer prevalent in the area, carried this

"new"[4] disease. Polly Murray was vindicated, but far too many in the medical community still brush aside Lyme sufferers with chronic symptoms and ambiguous test results.

Lyme is also far from "new." Not too long ago scientists found a five-thousand-year-old guy frozen in a glacier who they believe had the disease. Research suggests that Lyme in America dates back before the whole Plymouth Rock get-together, and that Native Americans were rife with the disease. When the white-tail deer was hunted nearly to extinction, and forests were cleared for farming and settling, Lyme disease nearly disappeared. Nearly.

Another theory of how tick-borne Lyme started doesn't date back that far. According to this perspective, it was developed after World War II in a germ warfare laboratory on Plum Island, the government-run animal disease research center that has long been rumored to have secret purposes. According to the theory, the disease was loaded onto ticks to be used as little biological weapons but something went wrong with containment. Plum Island lies two miles off of the eastern tip of Long Island and about twelve or so miles south of the Connecticut coast, not too far from the towns of Lyme and Old Lyme. Twelve miles as the crow flies or, as one conspiracy theorist puts it, "as the wind blows." *National Geographic* calls the Plum Island premise "compelling but controversial."

Just saying.

It was a guy named Willy Burgdorfer, a medical entomologist, who discovered the bacteria in the deer tick that causes Lyme disease. He was actually looking for something else but when he split open the tick under the microscope, he saw a little squiggly thing that looked like a fusilli noodle. The fusilli is called a spirochete and the virus it contains is called *Borrelia burgdorferi*, which sounds to me like an Italian version of Bergdorf Goodman, but it is in the business of only misery and pain. What's worse is it sells its wares from the shadows of confusion and misinformation.

The tests for Lyme in early 1990 were far from perfect and, if you ask me, they're just as archaic now. Accuracy in diagnosing and testing for Lyme disease has been one of the biggest challenges in the Lyme community to date. Being sick is bad enough, but being sick and not knowing why is insufferable.

I was about seven or eight years old when I started feeling the effects of my mysterious ailment, and it was more than just emotional outbursts.

On May 13, 1993, my sister Elizabeth was born, and around that time we moved back to Greenwich. My father's business was starting to soar and I think my mother didn't want us growing up too fast, becoming mini adults, which happens to many Manhattan kids. She has a wonderful maternal intuition when it comes to the well-being of her children, but even she couldn't see that I was being misdiagnosed.

We moved into an English Tudor on Mayfair Lane. On Sundays we went to St. Mary's Church on Greenwich Avenue for Mass.

Greenwich is perfect. It has to be: It's in the town's charter, I think. If you remember the movie The Stepford Wives you have a pretty good idea of what it was like to live in Greenwich. Everyone has their perfect houses, perfect fancy cars, and perfectly pretty children. The ideal Greenwich girl is tall and blond; excels at lacrosse, soccer, field hockey, or all three; wants to save the world; and is a wiz in math and English. Except for maybe wanting to save the world, I didn't fit into any of the Greenwich categories. Neither did my family. We were more like the hippies who made good and moved in down the street.

I was enrolled in the Connecticut chapter of the Convent of the Sacred Heart, which, like the one in Manhattan, is an all-girls Catholic prison…I mean school. My uncle Billy used to call it "Scared Heart"! My father drove me to school my first day and walked me into the building. Although I didn't know what the word meant back then, I had an awful lot of anxiety that day. I'd barely slept the night before. I also remember gripping my father's hand for dear life. When he let go, I began to wail. I'm not talking soft sniffles and drippy tears here, I mean full-out wailing.

Dad stayed until I calmed down. He introduced me to the third-grade teacher, Ms. Wilcox, who was really nice and promised to stay by my side and that everything would be just fine. She seemed pretty and friendly and somewhat familiar, so I cautiously took her hand and entered the classroom.

It was Ms. Wilcox who taught me a lesson that I remember to this day. When I began to get anxious at school she'd say, "Just let it roll off your back, like water off a duck!"

What I remember most about entering Sacred Heart was desperately wanting to belong, but feeling as though I didn't. I was the shortest in my class, didn't particularly like field hockey, and had dark hair. Three strikes and you're out! I thought everyone was smarter than I was. I went through the first part of third grade with a fixed smile, pretending I understood what was going on and not saying a word when I got confused. It was around this time too that I wanted to cut off my legs after gym class because my joints hurt so much.

I liked a few classes—drama and art were two of them. I also liked learning how to write in cursive. It was one of the only things that came easily to me. I would go home and practice it for hours, pretending I was a lady writing letters to my knight or prince.

I discovered that I could keep the fact that I was having trouble in school a secret for only so long—due to things called "parent-teacher conferences." After one such meeting, my parents took me to the Soifer Center for Learning and Child Development, in nearby White Plains, New York, where I was tested for a learning disability. I remember having to do memory games and put puzzles back together, neurological testing, three or four hours a day for entire week. I did that whole process twice. My nanny would drop me off at an office that smelled like coffee and was filled with toys and weird games. Here's how I remember doing one of them:

"Pick up the card and tell me what is missing from this picture," the therapist said as she took a sip of milky coffee from the lipstick-stained Styrofoam cup.

"The house has a chimney, windows, and a door, window panes, shingles…hmmm…Oh, I know what's missing! Green shutters and pink geraniums in wrought-iron planters in front of the door!" That's how every home in Greenwich, Connecticut, looked so I assumed that it was the norm for every house in the country.

"Well, yes," the therapist said, confused. "That is one way to see it. But look closer."

"You mean that it doesn't have a doorknob or weather vane?" I asked.

"Yes! A doorknob!" she said excitedly.

I rolled my eyes. *Duuuh.* I knew it didn't have a doorknob, but that was boring. I just thought that the test had to be more challenging than it was.

Besides having a hard time catching on with the little tests, I also found sitting in the same chair for more than fifteen minutes, let alone four hours at a time, to be painful. My whole body hurt. I was shifting around in my seat so much they assumed I was hyperactive, but then I would become so exhausted I'd put my head on the desk. The center's answer to this was to diagnose me with ADD and prescribe medication, which I refused to take. Granted, the rest of my family does have ADD and learning issues, so I was no different from them in that regard. I just had a pile of other issues on top of these that no one could put their finger on.

The ironic part of the whole ordeal is that tests revealed a rather high IQ.

High IQ or not, I just couldn't read. I had difficulty concentrating and remembering what I had just read. I remember being really confused because I had learned to read fairly quickly in first and second grade. Something had changed. I didn't understand why. I didn't spend time questioning it, however—I was in third grade, for Christ's sake! All I did was shrug and say to myself, *Well, I used to be able to read and now I can't. Guess I'm the dumb one in the class.*

My parents arranged for a tutor named Miss Brown, a tall, thin, waify woman, probably in her thirties, who was very kind and gentle. She taught me little tricks to do while I was sitting in class and unable to focus, like using index cards to guide me on the page when reading. She tried her hardest to make math and reading fun and creative for me.

I was probably the only one in my class who had a home tutor, which wasn't all that great for my self esteem, but I was grateful to have her and, later, Jody Sitver, who while I was in middle school guided me every night through my challenging homework, designed for advanced high school students. In Greenwich even third graders, it seemed, were on a college track, and usually the colleges they were on track for were Harvard, Yale, or Princeton. I kid you not.

Despite the fact that he's dyslexic, my dad also tried to help me with my spelling homework. For instance, to spell the word *finally* he would say: "*Finally:* fin, as in fish, and Ally is your name: fin-ally."

He said I should remember *fin* because I'm a Pisces. It was a good system, I guess, except for its limitations.

Between Dad's help and the tutor's, I did start to read a little better. When I got home after school, I would get a snack, visit my baby sister, Elizabeth, and read books like *The Baby-Sitters Club* and *The Boxcar Children* in her room while she played in her crib. It made me feel like a grown-up to be watching over her and reading. The stories enthralled me, and I felt content and happy lost in someone else's world.

Though my reading got better, not much else did. When the nanny would knock on my door saying, "Little Ally, morning-morning! Wakey-wakey!" in her giddy, bubbly northern Irish accent, I'd crawl into a ball and clutch the blanket. If I had been older and could have mustered up the energy, I would have tossed her out of my bedroom window.

I'd fantasize that I could airlift my bed, with me still in it, right to my classroom and then, as an added attraction, completely understand what the teacher was saying.

Instead, I'd pull the blanket over my head: Maybe no one would notice if I just stayed there and never came out. Maybe no one would notice that the teacher had to explain fractions to me again, and again, and again. Maybe no one would notice that I winced when I ran, or when I stood up after sitting for too long, or even when I was just standing for a period of time. Maybe no one would notice that my smile was a mask, that my vivacious personality was a ruse. Maybe no one would notice how much I hurt.

When I stood after sitting for a while, I'd wince from the pain like Nonnie, my seventy-three-year-old grandmother. How could an eight-year-old have the knees of a grandmother? And the gray wool of my school uniform skirt felt like sandpaper against the backs of my thighs and knees.

When I was around seven or eight my parents took me to Dr. Zimjhdmanashsnahdjks (that wasn't really his name, but that's how I remember it), a pediatrician. Dr. Zimjhdmanashsnahdjks was a bright gentleman, with two sons about my age. Though I have trouble remembering how to spell his name, I do clearly remember his telling me that he lectured his sons to always put their dirty clothes in the hamper RIGHT SIDE OUT! He said it like that, WITH EMPHASIS! Otherwise, he cautioned, they would come back to them folded inside out! I never quite understood why he was obsessed with this story, but he told it to me several times, and from then on, whenever I put my dirty clothes into my hamper or the washing machine, I always turned them RIGHT SIDE OUT!

Though Dr. Zimjhdmanashsnahdjks knew an awful lot, he didn't know squat about Lyme disease. He told my parents that I was experiencing a simple case of growing pains and probably strep throat. Of course! A bit more rest, stretching, and some hot pink liquid antibiotics that tasted like bubble gum were the solutions to all my problems!

This was around 1995, and Lyme wasn't exactly in the closet. It was out, and out in a big, media-covered way. People were concerned, and rightfully so. But the Lyme test on my tick had come back negative. What made a Lyme diagnosis even more remote for me was the fact that my mom didn't remember any rash. Doctors didn't know then that the red bull's-eye rash comes up in only about 40 percent of the cases and that laboratory tests on ticks can produce false negative results.[5] There was also the distinct possibility that the tick my mother took off me and had tested wasn't the only one that had bitten me.

So, for the next eight years I suffered through a maze of misdiagnosis, wrong medical treatments, and outright suspicion. The sore throats occurred on and off most of that time, the joint pain worsened, and my cognitive abilities declined.

It wasn't that I always felt bad, and that's the diabolical aspect of Lyme. I had some really great days, feeling like "myself" and happy, energetic, and pain/worry free. But those moments only made me feel as though I was lying or exaggerating about feeling bad. Sometimes being a little dramatic helped get my mother's attention. Unfortunately I wasn't clever enough to realize that my mother chalked up the theatrical explanations of the constant pain to my overreacting about something. She was constantly telling me, "Buck up, and get on with it."

My frustration got so bad something had to break.

It did. The "outbursts" that began on East Eightieth Street became worse and more frequent. I was angry, frustrated, and confused, and I felt disenfranchised. I believed people thought I was a liar and a fraud because no one could find out what was wrong with me. I felt as though no one was listening. My mom was my main target, and I made sure she heard me loud and clear. The outbursts came after Mom made me wear dorky clothes or kept me from going over to a friend's house. I would completely flip out. It was as if a force came over me that I couldn't control, as if a demon took over my being. It was scary, mostly for my parents.

For me? Well, it felt amazing! As if I were being released from some kind of nice-girl prison and could express my pent-up frustration, let loose, scream, and throw things. I could say mean things and hate everyone around me. Afterward, however, I would be left alone hating myself with the thought that I was just a bad little girl.

One of these outbursts came in fourth-grade math class. The homework assignment was sitting in my backpack, partly blank, partly scribbled on, and wrinkled. I had tried to finish the worksheet, had tried as hard as I could, but it was as if it were written in Chinese. My tutor hadn't been there the night before and my parents were useless when it came to math, so I finally gave up and hoped that my teacher, Mrs. Nolan, would understand.

When I arrived at school the next day, I knew I was doomed. I was the only one who hadn't completed the homework. I'd been in this situation before—I was the girl in the math class who was always raising her hand and saying, "Could you explain that to me again?" It always made me feel less than everybody around me. So, in that way this day was no different, except it was.

Mrs. Nolan was a young, happy, spritely woman and, for the most part, very kind, but she was also particular about things being done properly. My attempt at excusing myself from completing the assignment failed, and she sent me into the hallway. I felt like an idiot and a failure. My head was spinning with worry. How on earth was I going to advance from fourth grade? And if by some miracle I did, how would I ever be able pass the infamously tough Mr. O'Connell's English class in fifth grade? Would I be able to keep up and learn new material? I'm not sure if the anxiety I was feeling came from frustration and confusion or was a symptom of Lyme disease. It might have been both.

As if I wasn't worrying enough, Mr. O'Connell picked that exact moment to walk by me in the hall. When Mrs. Nolan peeked outside to see if I had worked on the blank worksheet, I snapped. I began yelling at the top of my lungs, accusing her of being a mean and awful woman. I declared that I hated her. I was red with rage.

I crumpled up the worksheet and threw it at her.

I imagine a lot of little girls experience anger, often toward their mothers. But looking back, I can see that much of my anger came from trying to deal with an illness I didn't even know I had. When I think back, I see this little human facing a world she just couldn't figure out. Why was everything so hard? I knew I wasn't stupid, and yet I felt as if I were. I knew I had pain in my knees, but everyone told me there was no reason for the pain. There's an old expression, "Feelings aren't facts." But good luck telling that to a kid who's eight or nine or ten years old. My feelings overwhelmed me until I snapped and checked out emotionally. I couldn't exist in the reality of those moments—it was too painful. So part of me would leave.

I don't blame little Ally one bit. Sure, the people in the path of my wrath usually didn't deserve it, and for that I'm sorry, but I am not at all sorry that the girl in the hallway with tears streaming down her face did what she had to do just to survive the emotional onslaught. The only thing that sucked was that I'd have to come back to reality, and when I did I was always disappointed. *What's going on?* I would say to myself when I'd return from the blackout the outburst provided. *It's still like this? Aren't you people listening?* In the moment, when my anger was volcanic and spewed from me like hot lava, I didn't even know why I was so angry and neither did anyone else. It was as if I were screaming from deep inside the volcano, *What's wrong with me?*

No one could hear me.

My actions might have come across as bratty or outlandish, but the truth is that I was quite the opposite of that overall. My parents definitely spoiled us in some ways but we were taught to have compassion and respect for people.

My parents also tried their very best to help me. They did everything to try to relieve the mysterious pain in my body. First it was weekly massages. Home massages were a luxury my parents were eager to provide; they had worked so hard to create a comfortable lifestyle for their family. Another luxury, and an unusual one for a ten-year-old girl, was visiting the chiropractor at least twice a week. Dr. Sharon Kaufman was as gentle as she was intelligent. I really loved talking to her because she took me seriously. I think she knew I was suffering from something other than what had been diagnosed, but she decided to focus on alleviating my pain. I think she knew that another blood test would probably not solve anything since I had had so many in the past years.

At the time of the math outburst we were living in the Hyatt hotel, waiting to move into Denbigh Farm, an eighteenth-century manor house in Greenwich. Dad's business was becoming successful beyond what anyone could have imagined—except Dad, because he always thought big. That day, when I arrived at the hotel my mother said she had gotten a call from the principal, who said I'd thrown something at my teacher. "Is that true?" she asked.

I crawled up in a ball and held my head. "Mommy, I can't understand math and she wanted me to do something I just couldn't do and she wouldn't help me. And I have to go into Mr. O'Connell's class next year and I'm scared."

I was just honest.

The rest of my memory about the incident and the time period surrounding it is pretty foggy. I remember watching *Anne of Green Gables* with Mom and seeing *Showboat*, a Broadway play. I remember too that Dad wasn't around much. He did, however, manage to drive all of us children to school every morning. But that's about all I remember from that time.

five

TO PEE OR NOT TO PEE

"Testing for Lyme may be misleading, as false-negative rates are as high as 60 percent in the first 2 to 4 weeks of infection."
—NATIONAL INSTITUTES OF HEALTH

Clothed in old-world preppy oxford shirts and khakis and wearing round, tortoise-shell horned-rimmed glasses and colorful bow ties, Mr. O'Connell seemed harmless enough, but it was his reputation, one whispered in the hallways, that made most students worry. "He is hard," it was said, the term used in the most unflattering way. That he taught fifth-grade English, however, brought on a special amount of angst for me.

Mr. O'Connell's reputation was not exaggerated. He would give spelling pop quizzes on the most difficult words you could imagine: *algorithm, photosynthesis, cryptic, rhododendron.* Nobody could spell them. It was fifth grade, for God's sake! The highest mark he gave me on one test was a 20, out of 100, and that's only because he gave credit for spelling my name right.

It wasn't only his tests that made him difficult. If girls were fiddling around with their shoes under the desk, he would have them take them off and put them on the railing on top of the chalkboard. I will say this: As tough a teacher as he was, and as much as I struggled in his class, some of his lessons on grammar stay with me to this day. So thank you, Mr. O'Connell, and may your participles never dangle.

In fifth grade, I had one set of friends from school and we became something of a clique: Courtney, Ana, Meryl, Kristin, Danielle, Alex, and Amanda. We did things together like shopping at the Gap, trying to sneak a look at *Cosmopolitan* magazine, painting our nails, listening to Mariah Carey, watching funny movies, making up dance sequences to music from the Spice Girls. The normal things twelve-year-olds of the day did together.

There was also the fact that my father was now pretty famous. Tommy Hilfiger ads filled glossy magazines and Times Square billboards. It's funny, though: I don't remember being aware of his fame. My parents, especially my mom, made a concerted effort to keep me sheltered from it. It was in school that I learned he was a big deal, when other students began talking about him to me.

A pattern began that would continue throughout my life: I didn't know if people wanted to be my friend because they liked me, or they really thought I was weird but wanted to be my friend because my father was Tommy Hilfiger. There are a lot of twelve-year-olds with famous fathers, and I'm not saying that my experience was any more difficult than theirs. But when you add the mysterious symptoms I was starting to feel, and the emotional insecurity that came with them, a toxic mix began to form that would be hard for anyone to withstand, let alone a fifth grader. All I wanted to do was be normal because I felt so different.

* * *

If Mr. O'Connell's class was a bummer, the summer afterward almost made up for it because of one specific incident.

In July I went with my best friend, Amanda, to Arcadia Camp for Girls, in southern Maine. One night we went to the boys' camp across the lake for a dance (such a cliché) and I started dancing with a guy who was tall, dark, and handsome, at least for an eleven-year-old. He had eyes with little hoods on the top like Leonardo DiCaprio's or Josh Hartnett's. Anyway, he was much taller and I remember him leaning down in slow motion to kiss me. We made out for what felt like two hours, in front of everybody. Such a crush! I remember going back and telling Amanda, "I kissed a guy! Oh my God! Oh my God! I can't believe it!"

Though I never saw him again, I've never forgotten the kiss.

The kiss across the lake opened up a whole world of possibilities for me. Throughout my life I've had some wonderful, compassionate, and caring boyfriends. In the short run, however, the magical kiss with the boy across the lake was the only magical kiss for a while. But next door to us at Denbigh Farm lived this guy who had braces and a crush on me. He would leave me little valentine notes in my mailbox, sometimes accompanied by a rose. The notes would read: "Meet me in the woods down the hill by the wooden bridge over the creek and we'll kiss." I guess I agreed to meet him because he was sweet, and I felt bad rejecting him (a people-pleasing pattern I am still trying to grow out of).

When the day came I was very nervous. I too had braces (and headgear, yikes!) and I asked my friends if I'd get stuck to him if I kissed him. I remember exactly what I wore that day: high-waisted, baggy jeans from the Gap, a button-up cardigan sweater embroidered with little flowers over a T-shirt, and brown suede hiking boots to complement my bob haircut, bushy eyebrows, and braces. Sexy.

We met by the wooden bridge and stiffly faced each other. "Ready?" he asked. I nodded "Okay, one, two, three..." It was about as romantic as a sack race, not the same as the kiss on the dance floor at all. I was so disappointed.

Things weren't much better in athletics. At an all-girls private school you're forced to participate in sports all year long: field hockey was in fall, basketball in the winter, and lacrosse in the spring. I was not good at sports. I was not competitive. It was not fun. I was so confused. In my disease-inflicted body I felt as though I were running in molasses while surrounded by cotton candy. But the good news is, I didn't give a flying fuck about sports. The only reason I participated was that I had to. I was the chick who would score a goal for the other team. The coaches would speak to us and I couldn't concentrate on what they were saying.

What I didn't know was that Lyme sufferers aren't cut out for the rigors of sports. One time I dropped unconscious, from what we assumed was low blood sugar. This was a feeling I would become very familiar with throughout my life, and one that is familiar to most longtime Lyme sufferers. There was another time I went away to squash camp in New Hampshire with Liz Meyer, a friend. I hated it from the moment I got there, and as I remember, Liz wasn't all that thrilled, either. Our first night I said how great it would be if something gave us a reason to leave the camp. The next morning I was in a fetal position in pain. Our moms flew up to New Hampshire in a small plane because I was in the ER with ovarian cysts (a common abnormality in Lyme sufferers). There was no hotel nearby for them to stay in, so they ended up sleeping on the floor of our dorm in sleeping masks and D. Porthault pajamas. That was pretty much the end of my squash career.

I did much better in drama and art classes at Sacred Heart. I was a pretty good painter. Once we had to pick a famous painting and try to re-create it with the material the artist used. I chose one of Van Gogh's *Sunflowers*. I did such a good job my mom put it in a fancy frame and hung it in our living room, right over the Duke and Duchess of Windsor's furniture (minus the chaise longue) in Denbigh Farm. An interior decorator once came to the house to take photographs for a book that was going to include Denbigh Farm and, thinking it was a real Van Gogh, took a photo of my painting, which they used for the book! I was ten years old.

By seventh grade I started to feel more socially at ease, but that comfort level had an unusual side effect. I would sit with my coterie of Courtney, Alex, and Danielle at lunch and we'd just die laughing. We'd be wearing our uniforms—blue and white pin-striped polyester cotton blend skirts with white Polo shirt—and someone would say something hilarious and I would laugh so hard I would pee in my pants. Literally, just as I did in the Piggly Wiggly when I was a kid. Spontaneous peeing became a bit of a theme for me. It was only later I would find out that Lyme disease can cause a whole host of bladder problems.[6]

At one point, Mom decided to take me to a urologist to find out why I peed when I laughed. She scheduled the appointment on Halloween. I went dressed in a black, stretch cotton evening gown, long white gloves, a pearl necklace, big black sunglasses, and my hair up in a French twist topped with a tiara. *Breakfast at Tiffany's*, one of my mother's favorite movies. My mother loves Audrey Hepburn, especially in her role as Holly Golightly. I walked into the appointment fully in character. "Do you mind if I call you Fred?" I asked the doctor as coyly as Holly Golightly said to her upstairs neighbor.

He gave me a pamphlet that explained Kegel exercises, which pregnant women do to strengthen their bladders, but I didn't do them because I was in sixth grade!

By seventh grade at Sacred Heart (the school had classes from first grade through high school) we had a very strict headmistress named Mrs. Hogan, who wore a lot of vintage Diane von Fürstenberg wrap dresses. She was all about manners and being "proper young ladies." We were made to study *Tiffany's Table Manners for Teenagers,* which I was forced to teach to my younger siblings every Saturday for one hour because I was the eldest, and put into a mothering role, and my mom was adamant about proper manners. At Sacred Heart, all that rigorous training made me feel as though I were in military school; we weren't even allowed to link arms with our friends in the hall. But I found a way to lighten things up.

Like my anger outbursts, laughter took me out of myself, away from the emotional and physical pain, but in a much more enjoyable way. That's probably why I let go the way I did (and do). I wanted to squeeze every bit of…well, juice out of it. When I was younger, my dad always made me laugh. He's really funny, and he can imitate anyone he's just met. He's also quick-witted. When Anna Wintour presented the Geoffrey Beene Lifetime Achievement Award to my father, she mentioned his talent as a mimic onstage and asked if he'd like to imitate her.

"Not to your face," he said.

I came to find that laughter had the power to transport me out of the pain and isolation that came with Lyme, but back before I knew I had the disease I laughed just because I couldn't help myself. I still do.

I love Cup of Noodles soup. I ate it almost every day at lunch. One day, when I was sitting with the same cast of friends, I laughed so hard I inhaled a noodle. I thought it went into my eye and I was still laughing but then I was peeing in my pants. I ran to Sister Shee-han in the lunchroom and told her that I had a noodle stuck in my brain. Luckily, Sister Sheehan was the cool nun—she used to tell us to pray in the shower because it was the easiest time to do it—but she might have overreacted to my situation. She put me in the front seat of her white minivan and tore up the pavement to the emergency room at Greenwich Hospital. They called my parents, who met us at the emergency room. The doctor poked inside of me.

"Honestly, the noodle is going to dissolve," he said.

six

VALIUM AND HELICOPTERS:
"ZE DOCTOR VIL ZEE YOU NOW"

"Don't tell me what I'm doing; I don't want to know."
—FEDERICO FELLINI

My mom and dad went out of their way to ensure there were outlets for my innate creative talents and I found that, like laughter, acting provided an escape from the cloud of Lyme disease that had begun to choke me. I took every extracurricular acting class in Connecticut, I think, and performed every chance I got. My parents sent me to acting camps both in Nantucket and at Stagedoor Manor in the Catskills.

My first night at Stagedoor, I was getting to know some of my bunkmates when someone asked me where I was from. I reluctantly told them Greenwich, which I hated to do because I always felt judged and categorized. Then one of the girls said that she heard Tommy Hilfiger's daughter was coming to camp.

"Really?" the other one chimed in. "I thought Tommy Hilfiger was gay." The rest of the heads around the room nodded. "He's a fashion designer, after all," one of them said.

I wanted to set the record straight and tell them that Tommy Hilfiger adored women, had four children, and was very comfortable in his heterosexuality—he was also very comfortable around others' sexuality, no matter what it was. But I thought discretion was the better part of valor in the situation. So I just kept quiet and waited to see how things played out. I eventually set the record straight and owned up to who I was. I am sure this might have embarrassed these people, but sometimes I liked to have a little fun and watch people dig themselves into the dirt.

At camp and in school, I acted in plays like *The Wizard of Oz* (I was the Lion), *Oliver Twist* (I was Oliver), and *Jack and the Bean-stalk*. At Stagedoor Manor we performed *The Good Woman of Setzuan* and I played an old woman. I took any opportunity to be involved with acting; it let me express the emotions and frustrations that continued to build within me.

As I look back on the character of the Lion from *Wizard of Oz*, I can relate to him more than I imagined at the time. Courage—that's all I needed. I can gratefully say that I found courage, not by visiting a wizard, but by digging deep down into the tunnels of desperation and blind faith.

When I was in eighth grade I got my big break. A family friend named Mary Pat Kelly wrote the book and lyrics for a musical called *Abby's Song,* a Broadway workshop production. The show was a Christmas story that posed the question, What if the shepherd boy in the Christmas story was actually a girl? Several of the roles in the play were young girls and Mary Pat thought that one—the lead's best friend—might suit me. I read some lines and sang for her and was cast in the role.

I was thrilled, but high hopes were almost dashed by my rigor-ous Catholic school. My rehearsal schedule was such that I would miss a considerable amount of time at school. Around that time, I went with my parents to Scotland, where they were going to renew their wedding vows. I remember being on a plane and reading something that, even with the new glasses my parents had bought me, was all blurry. I looked up from my book and began to plead my case. I wasn't getting anything out of school anyhow, I said. I couldn't keep up with the kids anymore. I was nervous about going to high school there. My parents knew how much I really wanted to do the play. To their credit, it didn't take too much to talk them into it.

For ninth grade I was enrolled into Eagle Hill, a school for children with learning disabilities, which I guess I qualified for, but the main reason I went there was that it was the only school in Greenwich that would accept me with the busy acting schedule. I suppose going there came with some type of stigma, but I never gave it much thought. To be honest, attending Eagle Hill gave me a lot of confidence in my ability to study and boosted my ego because, frankly, I could perform better than my classmates. Once again, though, I felt different and apart from the other kids. This time I was at the other end of the spectrum—I was the smart and well-behaved one in class. Still, my experience at the school was mostly positive and productive. The same, however, can't be said for my time during winter break.

My parents were skiers. We arrived in Lech, an Austrian ski village, at a darling little ski lodge hotel that was very quaint in a time-warp way. Elizabeth was only about four years old, and Kathleen was two. My brother and I were assigned a snowboard instructor and we hit the slopes as soon as we could go.

After getting warmed up and accustomed to being on a snowboard, I felt confident and cool enough to start trying to impress my attractive, blond sixteen-year-old instructor. My brother and I sat on the chairlift and were excited to practice our new moves and finally get a cup of hot cocoa. As we debarked the chairlift, I went to snap my foot into the board as fast as I could and prove that I had this down. While reveling in my glory of being all ready and waiting for the boys, I turned and the top half of my body fell to the left side while my legs stayed grounded to the board and *snap*! Something felt as if it broke on the right side of my body. I heard the pop.

I blacked out and woke up to the loud sound of a bright red medi helicopter landing in front of me. I was stripped down to my undershirt and the medics asked me where it hurt. I pointed to my right hip and cried. I was whisked up into the helicopter and injected with something that knocked me back out.

Meanwhile, down the slope, in a stone and wood restaurant with lovely views of the mountains, my parents were sipping rosé and eating homemade Austrian sausages in their Moncler ski outfits. Their blissful lunch was rudely interrupted by helicopter-roaring overhead on its way to the hospital one hour outside of the resort.

"Oh, I hope that poor person is okay," said my father to my mother.

Moments later a waiter dressed in traditional Austrian lederhosen approached my parents with a cordless phone, telling them they had an urgent call. My mother told me later her heart dropped and my father's face turned as white as the plate on which their now-cold sausages were sitting.

"Oh my God, where is she?" my father asked, holding his breath. When he looked back to tell my mother that they had to go to the hospital, she was already in the women's locker room removing her ski boots from the heating tubes, throwing off her white fur slippers, and packing to rescue her daughter.

Beige lipstick application? Check. Boots? Check. Are my two-year-old and four-year-old going to be okay if I leave to help my eldest daughter? Check. (They had a nanny.) Get Tommy to rent a helicopter to transport us to the hospital ASAP? No check. There were no helicopters available to leave at that hour. Driving in a tiny Audi in a snowstorm with a man who looks like he ate too many homemade sausages and who doesn't speak English? Check.

As I emerged from the MRI, I regained consciousness. German-speaking doctors and nurses in old-fashioned white uniforms surrounded me, explaining (in broken English) that "ze hip joint of you has slightly disclocate and zere is traumatic from your bones in zat area of your joints."

"I want my mom! Where is my mom?"

"I'm right here, sweetie. Don't worry, everything is going to be okay. Daddy is talking to the doctor. I love you." She turned. "Where the *hell* is that doctor? My daughter needs more drugs!"

A nurse brought a needle to inject into my IV. Warm. Calm. Dark. Sleep.

I learned later that my mother requested another hospital bed so she could sleep next to me. Beige lipstick? Check. Cashmere blanket? Check. Mason Pearson hairbrush? Check. Bergdorf Goodman pajamas? Check. D. Porthault cotton sheets? Nope. She went in anyhow. Roughing it! I can do this. It's happening. I woke and began to vomit from the strong painkillers they were giving me. "Get her a bedpan *now*!" I heard my mother yell. "She is throwing up all over! I can't stand the sight of vomit! Please give her something else! Oh this morphine, these doctors! Where are we? I can't have my daughter in this place! Where the hell is the doctor?"

A nurse in her white uniform strutted in as if she were coming to refill Mom's coffee. "Madam, ze doctor is at his annual New

Year's Eve party. He will be here in ze morning. May I offer you some Valium, madam? It calms ze nerves for you."

Did I fail to mention that this event occurred on New Year's Eve?

Waking up in a strange hospital in the middle of Europe on New Year's Day is like waking up in a dream—or better yet, a Fellini film set in the Alps in 1959. But it was 1999. The doctor finally graced us with his presence and my mother scrambled out of bed, ran into the bathroom to brush her hair, apply her lipstick, and slip her feet back into her Ferragamo bow shoes.

I, on the other hand, was puffy, pale, my hair a knotted, greasy mess. I had dried vomit crusted on my mouth and sheets, and I could barely see straight.

"Young lady, well, I am glad to say that today is ze day which you can leave only if you do zis one sing first wiz yourself for me."

"Okay, anything, I'll do it, tell me!"

"You must walk viz ze crutches from one end of ze hall to ze oza."

"Okay! Where are they? Mom, stop fussing with my hair! I have to do this so we can get out of here!" My mother put down the hairbrush and pouted at the sight of my hair, which she had attempted to conquer.

The nurse walked into the room carrying the crutches. Moving even to use the bedpan to pee was a challenge for me, so imagine my trying to get out of the hospital bed to walk. I believe they had given me doses of ibuprofen, since I could not tolerate the morphine, and I could feel a lot more. I felt as if someone were yanking my joint back and forth really hard. I had to make this work.

I told myself, *Don't be dramatic, just suck it up. Breathe, pretend you're that character at the end of the movie who is walking for the first time with her new leg and it is a miracle!*

Everyone was silently hunched over, staring, waiting, collectively hoping I could work the old-fashioned crutches.

One step, okay, fifteen more steps, don't put any weight on that right leg! Just lightly step and make it look like you're walking. One, two, three, one, two, three, one, two, three. I really don't know how much more of this I can do, and I have to take a break. Stop, breathe, don't cry, Ally, don't do it. Damn it, you're doing it!

Tears streamed down my face like rainwater off roses.

I was scared and felt very helpless, but the overarching feeling I had was pain. Shit was it painful!

I gave myself a pep talk: *Ally, you are used to pain, you can act your way out of this, you are strong, you are a fighter, a faker, a champion. Do one thing to make yourself proud. Now, come on! We can't have Mom making another scene, they will commit us both. Just do it.*

And I did it. Don't ask me how. When you really put your mind to something and feel that you have no other choice, some power comes over you and gets you through it. It's like a dream.

This determination and strength would carry me through some of my darkest times with Lyme disease. I had no idea that the power of my mind would conquer the uphill battles I was going to face in my future.

seven

THE GREEN LOLLIPOP EXCUSE

"Once inside the central nervous system, the organism (spirochete) can wreak all kinds of havoc, from memory problems, moodiness and depression to hallucinations, panic attacks, paranoia, manic depression, seizures and even dementia. Memory problems are the most common sign of a brain infection."

—NEW YORK TIMES

After I began to recover and returned home, I started rehearsals for *Abby's Song*. They were held in a space in the far west reaches of the Theater District in Manhattan, way off Broadway. Each day our driver would pick me up at home in Connecticut and take me into the city. At the time, I was feeling a lot of pain in my joints, especially my knees. I would sit in rehearsal on one of those taupe folding chairs with my jacket wrapped around my legs because they were so sensitive to the cold hard metal.

I had to use a cane at times because of the snowboarding accident, but luckily my mother had a fabulous collection of antique wooden canes with intricate handles. Truth be told, though, despite my pain and uncertain health I was happy to be out of my house and acting. I put everything I had into learning the lines and the role. I lived on protein shakes and peanut butter PowerBars in fear that I would have another embarrassing low blood sugar attack and have to stop the play. (The cause of these attacks still confuses me. I do know that other Lyme sufferers experience them.)

All of the cast's hard work paid off. We were an instant hit, first for a short run as a workshop production, and then for an off-Broadway run at City Center, a very respected venue with 1,200 seats. Paul Sorvino was in the cast and Randy Skinner, a well-known Broadway talent, was the director. The role I played was Lilly, the granddaughter of the innkeepers who turned Mary and Joseph away and the lead role's best friend. It wasn't the biggest part, but I hit one line every night that got the biggest laugh. I don't remember the line exactly but I do remember I channeled my inner Lucille Ball to deliver it.

One of the best memories of the show was when just about the whole Eagle Hill School came to a performance. My worst memory was dropping a line one night in front of a full house. I stood on stage frozen under the hot lights. There was a very scary moment but then a calm came over me. I remembered what they told me to do if this happened: I stayed in character and ad-libbed until the line came back to me.

Those days and nights of *Abby's Song* were really fun. Jackie Angelescu played the title role and Jackie and I became great friends. But there was trouble in the wings: In spite of the Scotland trip, my parents' relationship was on the rocks. There was a lot of tension in the air. I felt as if I was being forced to take a side, and my relationship with my mom was especially strained. Each night on the stage, however, I was free from all of the games, self-centeredness, and turmoil at home. Even though my knees hurt all the time and I often nearly passed out from feeling weak, I danced and sang my heart out.

I found out in Mustique that my parents were separating. My mother and I took a long weekend vacation there because I needed to get some rest and sunshine. I didn't have to be psychic to know something was going on: My father was constantly traveling and staying in Manhattan during the week. Still, Mom was shocked, I think, when I confronted her on the island, but also a little relieved. In a weird way, I was relieved, too.

Ignoring the secret had been stressful and awkward. Besides, most of my friends' parents were divorced so in one way it made me feel somewhat normal. Still, there was a time when the idea of my mom and dad not being together was unimaginable to me. They were nearly childhood sweethearts, for God's sake! They'd built a fabulous life and a family together as partners. They'd truly been in love. Though I might have been relieved that the secret was out, the news still left me in a state of sadness so deep I was numb. Mom made me promise not to tell my siblings, or anyone else for that matter, which was her usual method of dealing with anything: If you don't talk about it, it's not real.

In 2000, my father moved into the Trump International Hotel and Tower on Central Park West. I decided to move in with him so I could attend the Professional Children's School (PCS), a high school on West Sixtieth Street for the performing arts, a school for kids who were working mostly in the entertainment industry. Most of the students were in theater, the School of American Ballet, or the Juilliard School. It was not at all unusual to see someone playing the violin or dancing ballet in the hallway.

Moving in with my dad didn't exactly go smoothly. When I walked into the apartment for the first time I locked myself in the bathroom and couldn't stop crying. Richard and Elizabeth came with us to sleep our first night in the new apartment because it sounded like a fun, exciting adventure. But I stayed in the bathroom for a couple of hours and wouldn't let my dad in. I was traumatized at the notion that our family life had changed so dramatically, and that I was no longer going to live in the home my mother made for us. I was deeply saddened by the fact that my parents were no longer together, and that there was so much change in my life. I just wanted to go home, and Dad drove me back to Connecticut. I would move back in with him a couple of days later.

It was around this time that I started to experience acute anxiety and panic attacks. I didn't know, of course, that Lyme disease can invade the nervous system and produce mood swings, panic, obsessive behavior, sudden rages, depression, and other psychiatric symptoms. But I think it was also completely normal for the eldest of four children with separating parents to go through a rough bout with anxiety.

One day it really hit me. Chef Lynn Pasquale worked for my parents and watched over me while I was living in Manhattan and going to PCS when Dad was traveling for business. She had long, gleaming brown hair, and dressed very crunchy granola, complete with Birkenstocks. She was a ball of light and glowy happiness. Lynn and I became very close. We'd watch *Sex in the City* religiously, lip-synch and dance to Britney Spears songs, and giggle together all the time.

One day I was rehearsing for a play in school and felt particularly anxious. I chalked it up to everything that was going on with my parents, a blood sugar dip, and a cold I was battling. But on the short walk home I started to feel as though I was shaking apart. I remember standing on the corner of Sixtieth and Broadway thinking I wouldn't make it across the street without being hit by a cab or a truck. By the time I got into the elevator in my building I could hear my heart pumping, or at least I thought I could.

Inside the apartment door, the sight of me shocked Lynn. "Oh my God," she said, "you're white as a sheet!"

The last thing I remember is gulping for breath and collapsing into her arms. Lynn called 911, and when the EMTs arrived they took my blood pressure and said that if she hadn't called them, I might very well have had a heart attack and died. I don't think the guy was exaggerating, but it seemed a little extreme and scary. When they wheeled me out of the apartment on a gurney and through the marble gilded lobby of the gaudy Trump Tower, I was inclined to flip over and just hide my face. I was frustrated with my body for reacting so dramatically; I had no control over anything.

The doctor in the emergency room told me it was an anxiety attack. I was shocked. I didn't know anxiety could nearly kill you, and I certainly didn't know yet that Lyme disease could cause anxiety. These attacks would follow me throughout the next few years. I was prescribed Klonopin for a while by a fancy Upper East Side psychiatrist. After taking Klonopin on a daily basis as prescribed, I became a sloppy, sweaty, loopy mess. After a few blackout nights on that stuff, I tossed the pills and never went back to that doctor. I later learned that left unchecked, Lyme disease can cause permanent damage to the heart and even death by heart attack.[7]

I mostly liked going to PCS and made many friends there. I also started to do better in some classes, maybe because they weren't feeding me the traditional reading, writing, and arithmetic that

Sacred Heart served up. Ms. Sclan, the hippy English teacher who dressed like Miss Frizzle from *The Magic School Bus,* and Mr. Hart, the gay motorcycle-riding history teacher, were my favorites. They both respected me as a person as well as a student. Ms. Sclan assigned books like James McBride's *The Color of Water* and some of Shakespeare's most obscure pieces of work. Sclan also integrated film with poetry and literature. We watched Woody Allen movies and romantic comedies.

My teachers didn't realize that it was a miracle I could read and understand the books at all. All the work I'd put into reading, the remedial classes, the tutoring, and just trying hard on my own, had paid off. The same, however, could not be said for my math skills.

At PCS I was placed in the regular math class but it quickly became apparent that I was not at all equipped for what they were teaching. So I was switched to what was lovingly referred to as "the idiot's math class." Mrs. Moloff taught the class. At five foot one, dressed always in black, and with dark circles under her eyes, Mrs. Moloff was an insomniac who called an 800 number to help her sleep. For some reason, she was also obsessed with penguins. She had penguin posters, penguin pens, stuffed penguins, and penguin curtains. She was very shy and talked in a whisper. The class was so remedial I'm embarrassed to tell you about it. In high school I was doing multiplication tables. That's all I could understand! I just couldn't retain anything. They were trying to prepare me for algebra and calculus. I had as much chance of doing calculus as I had of building a Mars Rover.

My time at PCS marks one of the low points in my relationship with my mom. We hardly talked and since I was in New York and she was in Connecticut, we didn't see each other often—which was probably a good thing. I was mad because I believed my mother had left my dad, and because Mom had begun to tell me that I was overly dramatic when I complained about my ailments. I was annoyed because she always seemed to be too involved in her own life to pay enough attention to mine.

In her defense, she did have a lot going on. She ran Best & Company then, which sold luxury children's clothing in two stores, one in Greenwich and one in Bergdorf Goodman. She also had my two younger sisters and my brother to take care of, which consumed her. And she was going though a very emotional separation from a soul mate of more than twenty years. Those demands would have challenged anyone.

During this time, to help us bond my mom thought we should take a private acting class together. Maybe then she could better relate to me, the dramatic one. My drama teacher agreed to meet with us after class one day but, of course, I didn't show up. I showed very little respect to my mother at this time, but I did let the teacher know I wasn't going to come. You would think my mother would just then go home, but of course, she didn't. I can't imagine what my teacher must have been thinking, left alone with this woman he didn't even know in his classroom. I guess he figured he should make the best of the situation so he had my mother read a speech from a play. Mom put everything she had into it and the teacher told her she had a lot of potential. To this day my mother holds on to that moment as if she'd won a Tony. She makes me tell the story to strangers when we're in stores waiting on line. Every time she does I roll my eyes.

Maybe I was dramatic in some ways, but much of the drama I expressed came from years of frustration. In high school my health was deteriorating faster than any treatment could help me. My parents took me to famous sports doctors who treated me for arthritis.

At one point my father and I flew to Boston to meet a doctor affiliated with Harvard Medical School. He concluded from my blood work that I might have Lyme disease, but the tests were inconclusive. He told us the blood levels were just borderline positive. "It could be multiple sclerosis," the doctor said, which we'd heard before. Because of the symptoms I was reporting, from blurred vision to joint pain and muscle weakness, it was no wonder he suspected MS. When the doctor said it, my father's heart sank; his sister Susie battled MS her whole life and was bound to a wheelchair.

"But it is probably fibromyalgia," the doctor continued, "a disorder that is the most common musculoskeletal condition after osteoarthritis."

Somewhat relieved by the fact that 1) it most likely was not in fact MS and 2) I might actually be able to have a proper diagnosis and hopefully a solid treatment, off we went to a fibromyalgia specialist. I thought I had found the answer! We walked into a Park Avenue office and I was dressed like, well, someone not from Park Avenue. I had met my friends after school in Sheep Meadow, in Central Park, to smoke a joint. As I made my way to the office to meet my parents, I wondered if the doctor would be able to tell if I was stoned. I assumed that I wouldn't be the only one of his patients who self-medicated to ease pain.

"Why is your tongue green?" he asked when he examined me.

I guess I could have been honest and told him I'd just smoked some weed but instead I came up with a quick and stupid answer: "I had a green apple lollipop before I got here."

Maybe the excuse worked, or maybe it didn't, but he didn't say anything.

I left the office with medication to help alleviate the fibromyalgia symptoms. Anti-inflammatories, I think. They barely worked.

Some days I felt okay and on others I knew something was not right, but I hung on to the diagnosis because it was the only one that made much sense. Fibromyalgia actually included all of the strange symptoms I had been feeling. Plus, the diagnosis from a fancy doctor convinced my parents that I was actually experiencing the pain I'd been describing. Not that they thought I was making it all up; I just never felt they believed me all of the time.

In my mind I was halfway to real relief. Now all someone had to do was tell me what was really wrong with me.

eight

PAINTING, CHANTING, AND PITCHING FILMS TO FAMOUS ACTORS

"All that you need is in your soul."
—Lynyrd Skynyrd, "Simple Man"

It was in high school when a spiritual channel that I believe ultimately saved my life from Lyme disease began to open. Please know that I'm not saying this lightly. In my heart, I know I'd be dead if not for some of my spiritual beliefs. Lynn introduced me to a healer she used and I had phone sessions with her every week for a couple of months. She could not identify the disease that was growing in my body, but she suggested many detoxifying treatments such as salt baths to help with the symptoms I explained to her. She recommended meditation and vocal chanting. She knew my vessel was becoming thinner and thinner, I am sure. She knew I needed to do things to physically strengthen this vessel, but I was not disciplined or motivated enough to follow many of her suggestions. One suggestion I did follow, however, was tapping my third eye twenty-one times to relieve my anxiety. This actually worked well for me.

I had my first spiritual experience years before on Mustique, and I had always felt a spiritual connection to others. In high school, though, that connection matured to adulthood, so to speak.

At the time, I had a boyfriend named Garrett. We kept diaries together and wrote pages and pages about our enduring love, which lasted only about a year. He was a senior, I was a sophomore, and I went to the prom with him. Around this time, as I mentioned in the last chapter, I had been smoking pot pretty frequently. Along with liking the high like any other red-blooded American teenager, I found that pot helped with the pain in my joints and the nausea I was beginning to experience. The benefit of it outweighed the risk, I thought. In hindsight, I should have taken the healer's recommendations to help with the growing symptoms.

By then I already had a bad memory and was in a fog just about all the time. *What's the difference*? I thought. Besides, using pot was fun, and I was less angry and frustrated when I smoked it. With my friends, I would sneak off to Sheep Meadow in Central Park or to the park at Fordham University's Lincoln Center campus, which was across the street from my high school. There I would find relief and escape.

I knew that I could stop smoking pot anytime I wanted. At that time I'd become friends with a girl who didn't smoke pot or drink at all. When I began to hang around her I stopped drinking and smoking pot and instead turned my attention to a variety of spiritual disciplines: I read Buddhist teachings, attended chanting classes, and tried to stop smoking cigarettes ("tried" being the operative word).

The night of the prom, or in the wee hours of the morning after it, shall we say, Garrett wanted to go to a club on the West Side

Highway, and I didn't feel like hanging with a bunch of people getting wasted. So I walked home to my dad's apartment on Central Park West in my prom dress. At some point, I took off my shoes. I don't know whether it was my bare feet on the sidewalk or something else, but I had an electric connection to my surrounding that was maybe the most intense feeling I've ever felt. It was as though I had pure clarity and an awareness about myself and the world. I felt calm and centered. Happy.

Lynn was there when I got home. At the time, Lynn's cat was dying, and Lynn was distraught. I was able to put the event in a universal perspective that eased Lynn's pain. Even though I cannot recall the exact words I provided, I told her that her cat had probably offered her things in life that no human could provide. I told her that souls recycle and that dying doesn't necessarily mean the end, or never again. Death is just a transformation of the soul, a transition, and a part of life as an eternal continuous circle. In that moment, I could see how much I believed in fate, destiny, past lives, karma, and the fact that we all come to earth to learn lessons from each other. Even the souls of animals can teach us so much. I realized, too, that the insight I was able to offer Lynn could also help me on my own path through life.

I knew then there was an adversary within me trying to take over my body and mind. I didn't know it was Lyme disease, of course, nor did I realize how much more pain and torment it would put me through, but I knew I had to endure it to find out why I was given this path. I know this may sound crazy, but that night it was as clear to me as water in a mountain creek. I would come to find there was nothing crazy about it. The insight was real and it would ultimately save me: You have to go through Lyme to get through Lyme.

* * *

By the summer of 2001, my uncle Billy was dying of brain cancer. Besides being a musician, Billy was a landscaper and for a while planted the flowers and greenery on the roofs of many Park Avenue apartment buildings. It was thought that the pesticides that he used caused his illness. At the end he was in Los Angeles, and along with my whole family I went out to California to stay with him. He had just undergone his fourth operation, this one performed by a prominent surgeon whom Quincy Jones had recommended to my dad. The best in the world, however, couldn't save Billy.

Though Billy was still very ill, I returned to New York in the beginning of September for the start of school. On the morning of September 11, staff took us into the auditorium for an assembly. They announced that a plane had flown into the World Trade Center and some of the kids' parents had called to take them out of class. I went back to my Spanish class, where the principal told me my father had called and he wanted me to come home.

My dad had become quite close friends with Sarah Ferguson, the Duchess of York. I love Sarah Ferguson and I secretly wanted her to be my mommy (don't tell my mother). Once I spent a night at her house in York. That morning of September 11 she'd been interviewed on the *Today* show by Matt Lauer about her book, *Little Red*. She was scheduled to leave the show for an early meeting at a charity she was involved in but was running late. The charity's office space was on the 101st floor of one of the World Trade Center towers. The scheduling glitch saved her life.

My dad and I drove up to Connecticut and Sarah followed. New York was in shambles. Even though they were separated, my mother and father lived across the street from one another in Connecticut. My parents were and still are very close friends. My dad even had the same white fence my mom had in front of Denbigh Farm installed in front of his house so the kids would think of his place like an extension of home. We all spent the evening together at Denbigh Farm. Sarah slept in my bedroom at my dad's house. When I showed her to my room, I told her to wait in the hallway because I needed to check something.

At this point, I had picked up the weed again. Unfortunately the chanting and third-eye tapping was not helping my physical pain as much as I hoped. Pot was more instant and easy (and fun) anyhow! I wanted to make sure I didn't have any marijuana paraphernalia lying around my bathroom or anywhere else. When I finally let her in, she noticed a photo of herself, her two daughters, Beatrice and Eugenie, and me together on a vacation we went on one summer. Sarah thought I had gone into my room to put it there so she would feel special. I hadn't; the photo was one of my favorites that I kept around all the time. But I think what she believed made her feel cozy and welcomed, so there was no use telling the truth. She made me feel so comfortable when she had me as a guest in her home in England, and I wanted to do the same.

Four days after 9/11, Billy went into a coma in Elmira. He had returned to live with Nonnie after the surgery in Los Angeles to recover. We visited him and when I held his hand he looked straight into my eyes. I said, "Uncle Billy, I'm going to do everything in my life that you loved to do in yours. And you don't have to be in pain anymore." He squeezed my hand. That night he closed his eyes and never opened them again. Two days later they took him off life support.

After Billy died, I started to paint again. I hadn't painted since attending Sacred Heart. Painting became my therapy. The pressure of everything then—Billy dying, my health, my parents' divorce, and

9/11—was just too intense. I drilled three huge canvases together. I ripped photographs out of magazines, a lot of graphic images, a lot of images of targets, I guess because that's the way we New Yorkers felt then. I also ended up gluing a spatula on the canvas—don't ask me why, but it was probably some cryptic way of saying I wanted to scrape out all the icky energy in me and around New York. It was a pure stream of intuitive subconscious. I began to hear Uncle Billy's voice singing "Alexandria" to me.

My creativity in September 2001 was not planned or orchestrated. The only way I knew how to identify my emotions was through art because I had been so used to repressing them throughout the years. My art always held a deeper meaning, and I had things I was really trying to say. So I just dove right in and let it all come out. I would come home from school, throw on some sweats and a T-shirt, throw down a tarp, and just go for it. Looking back at the pieces I made back then, I can easily identify what I was going through as if I were reading journal entries.

I started wearing my hair up in a beanie when I painted because Peggy Lipton wore it that way. Peggy is the mother of my friend Kidada Jones, and one day we went to visit Peggy in the hotel where she was staying. I remember she looked so chic, so beautiful. Her hair was gathered up in a beanie. Peggy is a very centered and wise woman. We talked about astrology; she was spiritual, open, and soft, a very interesting person. And she listened to what I had to say. I remember thinking that I wanted to be like her when I grew up. She inspired me to be comfortable in my skin and to take care of my actual skin because I've got only one body!

I painted a lot of American flags then, but I'd make them very distorted. In one of the pieces I put strips of newspapers in the white stripes of the flag, and I wrote a long poem on the newspapers. It's funny how one thing leads to another. The poem opened me to writing. It was then I began to journal again. I didn't keep the journals every day but I began to enjoy writing little observances, short stories, and poems. I took a creative writing class with Ms. Sclan.

It's no coincidence, perhaps, that my spiritual awakening in Central Park coincided with an awakening of artistic urges. They both come through the same channel, I believe, and they came fast and furious. It was at this time that I began to walk the city with a video camera around my neck, and a few years later a Polaroid camera, taking pictures of things that I wanted to remember but was worried I'd forget. I put them on the wall in my first apartment. Those Polaroids became a kaleidoscope of expression and montage of my life. It was wonderful: I was an open vessel and the universe was pulsing through me.

It was around this time, my junior year in high school, that Dad told me about a screenplay our family friend Mary Pat had given him. Some years before, Mary Pat had written a book called *Proudly We Served*, about the African-American sailors aboard the USS *Mason* who fought German U-boats during World War II. Mary was (and is) a Northern Ireland historian, and the USS *Mason* was docked there during the war. "I've got a screenplay for you to read," my father said in the car as he drove me to Greenwich. "It's really cool, and I think it would be something you'd like." He was very excited about the project and wanted my opinion of it.

My dad always had a lot of faith in me when it came to my creativity. He trusted my taste in clothing and always brought me in to look at the designs of his new collections. He trusted me to make the right decisions about classes, which friends to hang around with, and how I wanted to spend my free time. He trusted me to navigate my own life.

On one hand, maybe Dad trusted me too much. I was his teenage daughter and yet he treated me almost like a very close friend. He loved me. That goes without question. He just perhaps let me grow up a little too quickly.

On the other hand, being my dad's daughter, and having my dad as a father, allowed me incredible adult opportunities that normal teenagers wouldn't even dream of, and one of those opportunities came with Mary Pat's screenplay.

I was flooded with ideas when I read the screenplay, and I wrote my comments right on the pages. My dad read them and thought they were helpful. I met with Mary Pat; we sat at the dining room table in our apartment in New York surrounded by all of my paintings. She explained how she got involved in the story, and how she knew all of the sailors, who were by then in their eighties.

My dad was passionate about the screenplay and said he'd finance it. I remember him telling Mary Pat, "We need heroes now." New York City was still an open wound from 9/11 and patriotic fever ran high. When Mary Pat and I met, I asked if she'd direct it, even though she didn't have experience as film director, and Mary Pat asked me to be the producer, even though I was sixteen years old. We figured that even though we didn't have experience, the story needed to be told.

You may be thinking, *Are you fucking kidding me?* How many sixteen-year-olds get such an opportunity? But I lived in a house of workaholics and if you weren't being productive and putting your best foot forward, you were just wasting your time, and no one cared how old you were.

I didn't give my age a second thought. I was just sure I could make it work.

We hired a casting director; I took the video camera that I always carried and put it on a tripod, and we brought actors in to read; we cast Kidada and her fiancé, Jeffrey Nash, who was interested in acting. Under my dad's recommendation, Mary Pat and I flew out to Los Angeles together and shopped the movie around, trying to get Hollywood involved. Sidney Poitier was Kidada's godfather, and I called him.

That's right. I cold-called Sidney Poitier.

"Hello, may I please speak with Mr. Poitier? This is Ally Hilfiger calling. Kidada Jones gave me this number to call."

A mature female voice paused on the other end of the line. Finally she said, "Please hold on, I will get him."

My heart was racing, my palms were sweating, and I was barely able to breathe.

"Hello, Mr. Poitier," I said. "I am very sorry to disturb you, but Kidada told me I had to call you."

"Oh, of course, Kidada. She's a great kid."

"Yes! Well, I am producing a film based on African-Americans being ranked in the navy during World War Two."

"Very impressive. Good for you!"

"Thank you! We are very eager to get this off the ground and hopefully get these war veterans the commendation they have been waiting for for so many years. We just need a big name to star in the movie. Are you interested?"

Holding my breath, waiting for the shoe to drop …

"Sounds really interesting, but I don't think I'm available," the Hollywood legend said.

After Mr. Poitier, the rest of my cold calls were cake.

* * *

Jeffrey Nash's sister is married to Forest Whitaker, and we went to the actor's house to ask him to play our lead. He also politely declined. We ended up casting his beautiful wife in a small role. When Denzel Washington was in Mustique vacationing with his family, my dad invited him and his family to our house for lunch. I didn't hesitate for a second to ask him. Denzel seemed shocked that a sixteen-year-old was pitching a film to him, but he was very nice and humored me. I gave him the script and told him about the movie, but he said he wasn't doing movies for a while.

I really grew a real pair swinging down there. What did I have to lose? The story had purpose. It wasn't selfish or vacant, and because of that I wasn't afraid. There is also something about a sixteen-year-old girl, a force like no other entity in this world, and I was accessing every bit of my teenage blind courage.

We ended up with a great cast. Along with Kidada and Jeffery, it included Stephen Rea, Aidan Quinn, and Ossie Davis in his last movie role. It was perfect.

Now all we had to do was shoot the damn film.

For three months we filmed in Buffalo on a destroyer escort naval ship that looked like the USS *Mason*. Three months in the winter, in Buffalo! We also shot interior scenes in Elmira for three weeks. During the drive up there, we got caught in a major blizzard on the highway, so we followed eighteen-wheelers that blocked the snow. My aunt Betsy had a Tommy Hilfiger outlet store in Elmira and gave us big, puffy down jackets to wear.

That was a special time for me, because I stayed with Nonnie. I would come home late at night and have the loveliest and coziest conversations with my grandmother about life. I would lie in my bed and on her way to her bedroom she would stop and say, "Honey, are you lonesome?" She'd come in and sit with me. She knew that things were difficult with my mom and that I wasn't always feeling well. I didn't have friends my age around me at all during the filming; I was among adults thirty years old and up. And I was to be considered their "superior" because I was the producer. It made things awkward, to say the least.

My joints were sore around this time but I sucked it up and trudged ahead—with a lot of weed to help me after the day was over. I hung out with the makeup, hair, and costume people and made friends with some of the extras. Because the story was about young African-American sailors, we hired a lot of young African-American guys from Buffalo when we were shooting there. As I was the youngest (by far) on the production side, it was my job to be the liaison between the cast and crew. Though stressful sometimes, it was a lot of fun. I loved meeting new people and having new experiences.

When we finished shooting in Buffalo, we went to Ireland to film a few scenes and my dad came along to help because we couldn't afford to bring our wardrobe crew on the trip. To dress the extras my father and I scoured the local salvage and thrift shops and dug through old garbage bags filled with moldy clothes. We didn't have enough extras, so my dad and I put on the smelly clothes and acted as extras in our own movie. (We used John Hume, too, the Nobel Peace Prize winner, who was a friend of Mary Pat's!)

In one scene, as an extra, my dad was handing out Guinness Stouts to the townspeople. I did the hair and makeup. We hired local women as extras. When they found out they were going to be in a movie they immediately went out and got their hair done. I had to redo all of their hairdos to fit the period. It was mayhem! I had bobby pins in my mouth, tape rolls around my wrists, safety pins stuck to my shirt, and combs in my back pockets. It was a role I'd play again in my twenties when I became a fashion stylist.

Though I have Irish blood from Nonnie's side of the family, it must not have been thick enough because I froze in Ireland, which made the aches in my joints almost unbearable.

Somehow we pulled it off. *Proud* opened in about ten cities. The film is far from perfect, but it's filled with the heart and soul of a project made with a higher purpose in mind. We got some very kind reviews and into at least one prestigious film festival.

Proud still lives and breathes, too. It's available on Netflix and is now part of an exhibit in the Smithsonian. Sometimes when I am flipping through the movie channels, I see it playing on Starz. It makes me feel—well, proud!

The summer after the release of the movie, I lived on Nantucket, wilded out, and partied way too much, but had the time of my life. I wanted to be a normal kid, but maybe my version of "normal" was a little off the scale. I hung out with college kids and fell in love with Led Zeppelin albums and listened to them with reckless abandon. I wanted to live in the 1960s and '70s, so I just pretended I did!

On Nantucket, I got a job working at a bikini shack shop on the beach. From when I was eleven years old, I had had summer jobs on Nantucket. I worked as a babysitter for a couple of different families, including for a woman whose mother was an editor at *Vogue.* I also worked in a beauty shop and for my mom in her store, The Children's Shop. At the bikini shack I was a great salesgirl. I was helpful and honest enough to gain the trust of the customers. I remember leading one mother of four kids gently away from the string bikinis and to the low-cut one-pieces. I also remember a very old and cranky gentleman with a young trophy wife who wanted four bikinis with different bottoms and shoes to match each outfit. The man told me he was in a rush and became very, very impatient with me. As I was carefully wrapping the merchandise in hot pink tissue paper, he began demanding that I give him the grand total of the transaction right away. Just my luck, that moment I had an attack of Lyme brain and my math skills went out the window. The man called me an idiot because I couldn't add properly. I felt like a big enough idiot as it was!

One of my coworkers rescued me and completed the transaction. I locked myself in one of the bathroom stalls and sobbed my eyes out. I knew I had made a fool of myself, and I knew that my brain was failing me more and more.

On Nantucket I also created, produced, and starred in a show on Nantucket TV called *In the House with Ally Hilfiger*. I got the idea for the show when I was staying with Kidada in Los Angeles. She introduced me to Cary Woods, one of the producers of the movie *Kids*. I stayed at Cary's house a couple of nights on his couch after eating too much Chinese food. He was awesome and we got along famously. He was the cochairman and creative officer of Plum TV, a cable provider that targeted wealthy communities.

He wanted me to have my own TV show on the network. *In the House with Ally Hilfiger* took its inspiration from the MTV show *Cribs*. I went to people's summer homes with a video camera, took a little tour, and asked questions like, "How do you decorate your house for the Fourth of July? What is your perfect outfit to wear to the beach while riding your bicycle? How does your home epitomize Nantucket? Why do you love it here? What is in your closet and in your garage?" I had a ball and I felt as if I was doing something productive for my future.

It would be an article in *New York* magazine that summer, however, that would have the biggest effect on my future. They interviewed me about being a movie producer at the age of sixteen, and the story they ran would open the door to a reality TV show—and some of the darkest months of my life.

nine

IN ANGEL'S WINGS...
AND HANDCUFFED

_"Many Lyme disease patients have acquired attention impairments
which were not present before the onset of the disease. There may
be difficulty sustaining attention, increased distractibility when
frustrated, and a greater difficulty prioritizing which perceptions are
deserving of a higher allocation of attention."_[8]

—ROBERT BRANSFIELD, M.D.

In the fall of 2003, I received a call out of the blue from MTV. Some
people there had read the _New York_ magazine article about _Proud_
and my role on the film as producer. The call was intriguing. They
wanted me to come in and talk about some ideas. They set a meeting
in their offices in the Viacom building in Times Square for October
31, 2002.

Halloween has always been one of my favorite holidays, and as
far as I was concerned, everybody should dress up in some sort of
costume. (I was still so childlike in many ways!) My friend Kate
and I decided to dress as a pair of angels. She was going to be the
naughty angel and I was going to be the good one. I wore a white

Dolce & Gabbana blazer with sharp shoulders, a flared, white canvas skirt with bustier, and brown crocodile stiletto high heels. . . . Okay, so maybe I was the nice but naughty angel. I also wore glitter on my face and angel wings. I thought I looked pretty cool.

I took a taxi to Times Square, climbed out, but then struggled to find the entrance of the Viacom building. For a little bit I wandered around Times Square in my angel outfit. Getting confused and lost had become an unwanted pastime, as my brain was not able to coordinate things very well, especially when it came to new places. You know those senile old ladies who walk around in shower caps in the middle of a grocery store? Yup. That's a safe comparison to what I was like. (When I wasn't in the middle of a Lyme flare-up, I was pretty good at directions and getting places.) I was not being treated for any of this brain fog. At this point, I had no perspective on how or why I was deteriorating so rapidly. I formed a kind of acceptance around the fact that I was unable to function normally both physically and mentally. I also hid it from people the best I could, and acted my way out of it. I didn't want people's pity, I wanted answers and solutions that were apparently impossible to attain. I do remember being in tears a few times during high school with excruciating joint pain. The principal in my school was supportive and helpful in trying to offer solutions to these ailments. She recommended doctors and allowed me to leave in the middle of the day if I had a migraine or to see a doctor who ultimately would not do anything for me anyway.

I finally figured out how to get in the Viacom building and walked inside, where I saw a very tall escalator. It seemed to climb to the clouds. At the top of it, a woman with chin-length light red hair, a milky complexion, and a warm smile waited for me. She introduced herself as Wendy. Wendy was just as warm as her smile. I remember thinking that she must be from the Midwest. She led me to an office that was filled with lots of toys, like Beanie Babies, stickers, and other random items.

There were also two other people in Wendy's office, but I was so nervous and fascinated with the crazy explosion of colors and stuffed animals everywhere that at first I failed to take notice of them. Once we were introduced, everybody was very nice. They asked me about *Abby's Song,* about *Proud,* and about the television show on Nantucket. "You're so young," one said. "You're so interesting," added the other. "You have such a great personality." And then Wendy said, "You'd be great as a VJ for us." *VJ* stood for video jockey, the on-air talent who hosted the music shows. It was a big deal.

At this point, any other seventeen-year-old kid would have been thrilled. But I pictured myself with a microphone, talking about celebrities I knew nothing about, and I said, "I don't really think that's for me."

I know I'm running the risk of sounding egotistical, but I just didn't think being a VJ was very meaningful. I didn't feel it at all. My reaction to the offer drew some semi-stunned expressions. There were a lot of open mouths in the room. Along with being ballsy, I'm also the consummate people-pleaser and there are moments when the combination of those two character traits is creatively combustible.

So I said in a kind of open-ended way, "I'd be interested in helping you guys create a show." I half-expected my statement to land with the thud of a September issue of *Vogue.* Instead, it piqued their interest.

"What kind of show did you have in mind?" they asked.

At the time, I was at my zenith of social awareness. I was deeply concerned about changing the world. I was into my throwback hippy phase. I often wore my dad's old cargo pants, smoked pot, and listened to Crosby, Stills, Nash & Young and Led Zeppelin. The persona I'd developed was as far away from my preppy upbringing in Greenwich, Connecticut, as I could get.

I was also in a full medical, spiritual, and creative counterattack against the mysterious illness that caused me so much grief and pain. I remember not sitting down much in Wendy's office because my hip joints were in a constant state of inflammation. In the fall, with all of the mold in the air, my autoimmune symptoms flared up. In Lyme patients, mycotoxins, or mold, can cause coughing, wheezing, memory loss, confusion, brain fog, and cognitive impairment bind.[9] In the middle of the meeting, due to my joint pain, I walked to a window that overlooked Times Square. They must have thought I had some chutzpah. Who walks around someone's office during a meeting? In a full-blown angel costume? What kid turns down a VJ offer from MTV? Who comes to a business meeting dressed like Adam Lambert in the afterlife?

But I could see they were intrigued. They asked me to come up with some ideas for a show, and I think they expected me to go home and return two weeks later. Instead, ideas flowed out of me like mudslides during El Niño. I was relaxed. Fearless. Inspired. I didn't need MTV, I thought. But maybe from their perspective I was a glimpse into teenagehood, which was their main demographic. This burst of creativity and flurry of brainstorming led to a more focused idea.

I thought the lives of private school kids in New York were really interesting—or very unusual. We're like mini-adults, I said; we go to all these fancy stores, restaurants, and clubs and we are very, very independent. Wouldn't it be interesting if we showed all of these kids acting like adults, doing fancy adult things, and living this fast-paced life while also dealing with normal high school issues? Issues like who you were going to take to the prom, what you were going to do after you graduate, how you were going to get through the SATs.

In spite of our independence and privilege, I said, we were also dealing with issues such as neglect from parents, being raised essentially by nannies, suffering from prescription drug addiction, eating disorders, and intense emotional turmoil. Some kids who went to those beautiful schools were living totally unhappy existences.

What made it worse, I told them, was that no one took us seriously. I was so tired of people having preconceived notions: "Oh, you have all this stuff and live this amazing life," they would say. "How could you ever be unhappy?" What they didn't know was that behind those closed doors were some of the most painful and lonely realities. I wanted people to stop criticizing these kids so harshly. Were some of them spoiled? Yes, but being spoiled doesn't stop kids from having very dark lives and, in fact, privilege sometimes makes them even darker.

I told the MTV reps I wanted people to stop judging the book by its cover and instead go deep into the pages. What I didn't tell them, and what I would never tell them, was that my own pages contained a private torment. I was sick much of the time and had seen countless doctors. What made it worse was that no one could tell me what was causing my pain, which made many doubt I even had any. My parents were separated and I was still intensely grieving Uncle Billy's death. These were the issues that fired my motivation.

I knew I couldn't create a show on MTV focusing on the fact that one in fifty American kids were homeless and starving.[10] So I said, "The kids in the privileged one percent yearn for their mom and dad to pick them up after school. They long to have breakfast and dinner with their families."

In the office, heads nodded as if they were rocking out to Jefferson Starship. I was on a roll.

"Maybe we could also have a camera crew follow a bunch of kids in some rural town in the Midwest," I said, "and see how the two groups compare and contrast, to show the parallel story lines." That was a naïve moment. I don't think MTV was in the stereotype-breaking business, or that they gave a hoot about the private torment of rich kids or poor ones in rural America. But I think they saw the possibility of a hit show.

Not too long before, two very successful movies, *Clueless* and *Cruel Intentions,* had played on spoiled rich kids themes. I can see now that MTV had no desire to go any deeper into the issues behind that kind of glitz and glamour. But they liked my name, and the fact that I brought more than an idea and a Chanel bag to the table.

They didn't say any of that to me, of course. What they said was: "We love the idea! Can you please write a treatment for us?"

"Be glad to," I said, and they set up a meeting for the end of the following week.

When I walked from the office I could have flown with my angel wings. Not even the fact that I had real difficulty stringing a coherent sentence together, let alone not knowing what the hell a treatment was, could take the air from beneath me. I'd find a way. I knew from my experience with *Abby's Song, Proud,* and *At Home with Ally Hilfiger* that I'd be able to pull it off.

As soon as I took the escalator down to the street, I called a close high school friend. Jaime Gleicher was a great actor and very smart. I knew she could write the treatment, whatever it was. I knew she was the perfect one to help me. I then drove home to Connecticut. I had a tradition of taking my youngest sister, Kathleen, trick-or-treating in Greenwich and Bedford, so I wanted to get back on time.

I met Jaime at Fred's for lunch the next day. Middle-aged women with facelifts surrounded us, some carrying the same Prada bag and wearing fur vests that they slung over the backs of the wooden chairs. Fred's is on the ninth floor of the Barneys store on Madison Avenue and is sort of a ladies-who-lunch, power-tie kind of restaurant with an insanely good chopped salad. I'd told Jaime about the MTV meeting and the treatment they wanted me to write (somehow I figured out what a treatment was), and she was very turned on by the whole concept. Jaime and I were interested in the same issues. We were aligned in that way. Often we had philosophical, spiritual, and intellectual conversations. I really liked her company.

At lunch we were supercharged. Ideas flew across the table. Jaime furiously took notes. Although I was excited, I felt insecure about not being able to recall words, not being able to explain things well. Thank God for Jaime. I was deep into Lyme brain. I was ashamed even to tell Jaime that I felt so inadequate. I just said she was a better writer than I was and could describe the concept better on the page.

I can't remember when we began to write, but I do remember standing behind Jaime as her fingers flashed across the keyboard. The pitch was centered around Upper East and Upper West Side privileged kids and the real issues that existed behind their closed doors. We wanted to highlight normal teenage issues that every other kid in America and in the world was facing, but with New York City as the backdrop. We came up with rough ideas for some of the episodes.

The next week, Jaime and I went back into the Viacom building to meet with Wendy and the other MTV people. The tenor of the meeting had changed somewhat from the first one. Things were a little more businesslike and serious. They were still nice, but right away they started firing questions: "Where do these kids shop?"

"Where do they go at night?" "How do they get into clubs?" When I told them that they'd either know the bouncer or have a fake ID, you'd think I'd just handed them Madonna's teenage diaries.

Truth of it was, I wasn't as savvy as I seemed.

About a month later, on Thanksgiving eve, I went with my friend Kate to a hole-in-the-wall Irish bar in Katonah, New York, a bar as far from Manhattan's trendy Meatpacking District, now known for its clubs and boutiques, as you could get. I had just acquired a killer fake ID from the back of a cheap clothing store in Greenwich Village, but the name I used was Alexandria Cirona. I thought I would remember my mother's maiden name better than something I made up, what with my Lyme-y brain and all. Our IDs worked like a charm and the bouncer let us in. (Truth be told, I think they let anyone in who could see over the bar.)

Inside the place was dark, crowded, and a little seedy—perfect for a seventeen-year-old. We sat at one of those high, circular tables right in the middle of the room. There we met one of Kate's friends, who went to the bar to get us all rum-and-Cokes (rum-and-Coke was my first drink ever; I'd had it on Mustique), but before I even had a chance to take my first sip in came the cops. "Are they looking for someone?" I asked Kate. I was so naïve.

Along with being a big party night for kids, Thanksgiving eve is also a big night for police to check on underage drinking. When they came to our table and asked for IDs, I don't know what was racing faster, my heart or my head. I didn't know whether to show them the fake ID or my real one. Of course I couldn't remember what name I used after all, and I also knew I couldn't lie. I just can't.

It didn't matter which ID I showed. The cops immediately knew we were underage and a female cop asked us to step outside. It was freezing cold and I was wearing a puffy vest and a sweatshirt. I thought they were just going to give us a ticket and tell us not to go back into the bar. When they told us to get in the back of the cop car I blurted out, "Wait, what?" I really didn't understand the intensity of the situation.

I remember nervously giggling. I was taking acting class and decided I could use the experience as some kind of tool, so I might as well just get all I could out of it. Kate was an actress, and she felt the same way. When the cop car pulled around to the front of the bar, I cheekily asked if they were going to put handcuffs on us.

"We weren't going to, but if you want them . . ."

"Yes! We want them! We want our heads held when we duck into the car, everything!" It was as though I was ordering the deluxe package at an amusement park. The officer even thought it was funny and was laughing as he slapped the cuffs on me. Well, "slapped" might not be the proper verb. The cuffs were so loose we could pull our hands out of them. In the back of the cop car I inquired about our Miranda rights and was assured we'd get the full treatment down at the station house.

When we got to the station there were two fellows from the same bar in a separate cell who looked miserable, as if they were coming down from their buzzes and just bummed the fuck out. Kate and I hadn't even sipped the first drink we had ordered, and we were excited like two giddy idiots. When I posed for my mug shot I asked if my hair looked good. I helped the cop fingerprint me and made friends with the other officers.

I had a moment of terror, however, when I saw them going through my bag. I thought they might find a half-smoked joint, a nugget of weed, or rolling papers. They didn't, but they did find my fake ID. When they booked us, they put down "Felony D" on the form. "Oh my God!" I exclaimed. "I'm a felon!"

The female officer put Kate and me in separate cells and offered us water, blankets, and ham sandwiches. "Water would be terrific," I said as if I were ordering a cappuccino. Then I lay down on the bench and took a nap. We had to wait for the judge to get out of bed and to the courtroom.

When he arrived, the cop attached Kate, the two bummed-out boys, and me in ankle cuffs and marched us like a chain gang into court. I felt like a badass rebel living the nitty-gritty. The judge was really grumpy and made us feel bad by saying, "You should be ashamed of yourselves! How do you think your parents are going to feel?" One of the nice policemen, however, gave us a ride back to our car.

The next day, for Thanksgiving, my family went to Nonnie's in Elmira. When I saw the look of shame and disappointment on my father's face I felt guilty, however, so I retreated onto Nonnie's couch and curled up to sleep. The worst of it was letting my parents down in the middle of all of their troubles. Later on, a defense attorney who was from the same hometown as my father managed to have the charges reduced and the record sealed.

Though Jaime and I were acting savvy in the MTV office, and all the television execs were very excited about the prospects of the show, I was worried. All I could think about was that the cool clubs where wealthy kids hung out were not going to allow cameras to record them serving underage kids. They would have been shut down, and I would have been partially responsible for ruining people's livelihoods. I thought, *No way is this whole thing is going to pan out. It's impossible.* But while I was thinking that, the MTV reps were saying, "We want you to shoot a pilot. Get some people together you can follow to a club, and highlight the lives that are more unusual."

My head was spinning trying to think of whom I could ask to film. I was already sorting out different locations that would depict this glamorous life in the best possible way, while showing the real issues that were happening. *How can I get places to let us film in them? Will my friends' parents even allow their kids to take part in such a thing? How many camera crews? What is the budget? How many kids will we need to wrangle? How many guys? Girls? Do they have to know each other? Well, probably, because we'll need some dynamic drama.*

Spinning, I tell you.

We started calling all the people we thought would be a good fit for the show. Finding them wasn't difficult at all; the Professional Children's School was full of privileged Upper East and Upper West Side kids, most of whom wanted to be actors. It was the perfect talent pool. I remember calling one guy who had a sexy, bad-boy, drinks-martinis-in-the-middle-of-the-day vibe, exactly like the Ryan Philippe character in *Cruel Intentions*. Pretty quickly, three or four kids from PCS agreed to be filmed for the pilot. When we arranged for a camera crew we were set, except for one small problem. The night before we were going to shoot, our on-air talent began to bail, one right after another, until we had no one. The excuses ran from "I can't go because I have an audition" to "I have to go to the country house with my mom."

We were screwed.

As I remember, the pilot was supposed to show the kids getting a limo, getting a room at the St. Regis hotel, going shopping, and eating at Cipriani; after all that they would go to a club. What really happened was Jaime and I got the limo, we got the hotel room, and went shopping at Henri Bendel, but when it came to going to the club I was just too exhausted. Luckily, the shooting schedule didn't include the camera crew following us to the club. Instead they were to film us the next morning at brunch, where we would recap the night before.

The next day, over mimosas, Jaime and I made up a night at the club in front of the camera. I talked about "Jason" and "Michelle" hooking up, how crazy it was, and can you believe how messed up Bridgette got? Meanwhile, I actually had been in bed by nine thirty with a fever, which I seemed to get every night and which had been getting worse over the past weeks. I thought the crew would know I was lying and how Jaime and I had screwed up, and I thought there was no way MTV would pick up the show.

Wendy called for another meeting pretty quickly. When we went back to her office, she told us that the head of MTV had greenlit the project and wanted us to begin production right away.

Right away? *Right away?* I thought I'd have more time to think things out, maybe even bail if I wanted to. Welcome to the world of reality TV.

The big news, however, came with a big condition: Jaime and I had to be the stars of the show.

"Wait, what?"

Apparently, they liked our on-screen energy.

My heart dropped to the bottom of my stomach. My red flag shot up, and my every instinct was yelling, Stop! I was very scared. It felt so weird. First of all, I didn't think I could physically hold up for a season of shows, let alone deal with the whole privacy issue. We were actually a very private family. I'd been sheltered my whole life. There were many occasions when prestigious magazines wanted to come to our homes and include us in the photos, but my mother refused. It wasn't safe or appropriate, she thought. My parents didn't believe in exposing our family for the sake of publicity. I shared the same beliefs, or I thought I did.

I remember clearly thinking, *My mom is not going to like this one bit.*

I was right.

ten

DEAL WITH THE DEVIL

"Do not get attached to worldly things and pursuits.
Be in the world, but do not let the world be in you."
—Sai Baba

As I mentioned, I believe in reincarnation. If I had a choice I would come back as a tree. Beautiful and majestic oaks, maples, and pines surrounded me when I was growing up in Connecticut. At summer's end, Greenwich begins its transition to a Van Gogh painting come to life. If you haven't seen it, please come. Words do not do justice to the beauty of the Connecticut fall.

But what I like most about trees is not the colorful leaves or the soaring heights but the long, deep roots that anchor them to the earth. Trees are solid, grounded, and strong. They rejuvenate, shed the old, and grow new fresh leaves. They provide oxygen, food, and shelter, among so many other things. Their roots remain in the earth long after they have gone.

Shel Silverstein's _The Giving Tree_ has always been one of my favorite books. Reading it makes me wonder why humans are so selfish and unable to give back to the majestic trees as much as we take from them. If humans gave half as much to nature as our precious trees gave us, our world would be a more magnificent place, don't you think?

On Denbigh Farm we have a giant fir tree. My mom's property is one of the highest points in Greenwich. For one Christmas, she surprised us by dressing the entire tree with colorful twinkly lights. You could see them all the way from North Street in town.

Maybe that's why I love trees so much. If I am ever feeling empty, lost, insecure, or disconnected, I gaze at a tree and visualize that I have my own roots connecting me to everything in the world. My mother is a major tree hugger—literally. She will hug a tree and identify what kind of vibrations the tree holds. I have become the same. I hug trees and feel them breathe. There were many times in my life when I wished I had someone to stop and hug me, and feel me breathe . . . or to tell me *to* breathe.

For example, when I joined MTV.

When I told my dad that the TV show had been green-lit he was ecstatic. "You're going to create, produce, and star in a national—international—show for MTV? This is awesome!" I've always trusted my dad implicitly, and I knew he would never be excited about something that would be bad for me. Besides, my dad knew a good business opportunity when he saw one. "You don't ever want to live with regrets," he said.

It did feel exciting to me, and I'm not blaming my dad, but part of me felt like I was the princess in Sleeping Beauty, being led to the glowing spindle. Any time fear set in and I wanted to turn into my forest to sing with the animals and trees, I was called back with the cursed lullaby of that spinning wheel. It was glowing, warm, inviting. *Come, child, come and touch the wheel and all will be well,* said the witch behind the wheel. The show was the spindle and there weren't many people telling me to run. Everyone around me seemed caught in the same spell.

After talking to my dad, I went over to Jaime's apartment on the Upper West Side. "Listen," her mom said, "this is a really great opportunity. It could lead to so many things in your careers." I liked acting enough and I guess I was pretty good at it—I even found a commercial agent to represent me. I wasn't exactly over the moon at the prospect of doing commercials for laxatives or feminine products, however, and I hadn't completely thought out any other long-term acting plans. I knew I wanted to do film. I thought I would be good as a comedic actor. The truth was, though, acting was difficult for me in some ways because it felt inauthentic, and I didn't like having to be deceptive to succeed.

I was also frightened to death of going to college. I barely got out of the idiots' math class—how could I survive a college curriculum? My parents and I looked at Eugene Lang, a liberal arts college and part of the New School, in Greenwich Village. I wanted to study writing and producing, but I was so worried that my brain function was deteriorating. I thought I was getting dumber. My vision was a problem. My ability to retain information and repeat anything I had learned was a problem. My ability to focus was a problem. I knew that going to college would only magnify all of my learning issues. Although I didn't know that Lyme disease was causing all of these problems, I did know for certain that those problems weren't getting any better. In fact, they *were* getting worse.

Some of my ambivalence about career direction also came from being my father's daughter. I had this huge presence in my life standing on the pedestal I had built for him, a person who had achieved so much acclaim and success. How was I supposed to stand on that high platform next to him? I'd already heard the whispers, or had I imagined them? "Is she as smart, as talented, as creative as he is?" I was reluctant to work for my dad because I didn't want to hear people say, "She's only here because she's his daughter." "I bet she doesn't *have* to make any money." "No matter how good she thinks she is, she'll never get close to her father's level of success."

In being Tommy Hilfiger's daughter I reacted to opportunities in one of two ways: I'd either run up the white flag and say, "Fuck it, what's the use?" or I'd work my tail off to prove myself worthy. This added to me wanting to deny the symptoms I was experiencing and hide them from people. I didn't ever want anyone to think I was shirking work or anything like that. I had worked so much to prove that despite the money, I still had a work ethic.

So when Jaime and her mom began talking about how we could actually help teenagers, and how it was an opportunity to shine a light on real issues on camera, I began to think that maybe this was something in which I could become totally invested. Maybe there could be a higher purpose to this. *Sure, some of the glitz and glamour will have to be there, but we really might be able to help kids. We have issues and we can talk about those issues.*

Maybe we can actually do something good.

By the time I left Jaime's, I was convinced I was about to embark on a great and meaningful TV show. You may be snickering. *Please,* you're saying, *how could someone ever be that naïve? Reality TV dealing with important social issues? No way!*

You have to understand that there was nothing with which to compare our show. The Kardashians were years away; Real Housewives wasn't even an idea yet. Reality TV had not yet exploded in popular culture. The biggest reality show on TV then was *The Osbournes,* which, as I'm sure you remember, followed the rocker

Ozzie Osbourne's family. *"Sharrrron!" The Osbournes* was a huge hit for MTV and sent TV execs scrambling to come up with similar ideas: Paris Hilton and Nicole Richie's *The Simple Life* for Fox was in production right behind us. No matter what you think of reality TV, it was a phenomenon that changed the television medium forever, and our show was on the leading edge of that cultural shift. We were in uncharted territory.

I started to become excited, feeding off the energy around me—I just didn't realize that it was negative energy. I put my producer's hat on. I felt the way I had when we made *Proud*. I was going to put everything I had into this show. I was going to make it on my own.

Seventy-five Rockefeller Plaza looks like something right out of an Ayn Rand novel. It has an all-marble entranceway and those old-style elevators painted in a gold leaf. We were there to sign the contract at the office of the lawyer to whom my father had introduced us. Jaime and I arrived without a guardian, manager, or agent. As I remember, the MTV people were a bit surprised by that. In fact, I never went to one MTV meeting with anyone other than Jaime.

As we were ascending in the gilded elevators to the lawyer's offices, I had a feeling in the pit of my stomach. It was the feeling you get when you know you're about to do something dangerous. But I also felt that it was too late for me to turn back. Jaime was very excited, and so was my father. I thought it would be so spoiled, bratty, and stupid of me to walk away from an opportunity that many people would kill for. My heart was pounding as we reached heavy glass doors of the lawyer's office, which had huge windows and was brightly lit.

When we entered the office, the thick contract lay on a mahogany table. I'd tried to read it and could barely understand a sentence.

I knew that our lawyer and the MTV lawyers had gone back and forth for weeks trying to get it in tip-top shape—at least that's what I was led to believe. I was not privy to any of the negotiations. No one had actually even explained the contract to me in layman's terms.

In the office, I remember asking whether we would have any control over the editing process, and we were promised that we would get to see the dailies and rough edits and have some input. There was a clause in the contract about merchandising and I was told that MTV had control over all merchandise, from bobbleheads to board games. Though it didn't seem fair, the thought of having a bobblehead doll of me did make me giggle.

I remember asking how we could get out of the contract once it was signed.

"You can't," our lawyer said. "You're legally obligated to allow them to air however much they have filmed."

Jaime and I, of course, wondered how much we were going to get paid. Our lawyer prefaced his answer by telling us he'd worked hard to get the number up to where it was and that the "number is a good one. Trust me," he said.

"Is it as much as the Osbournes get?" I asked.

"Not a good comparison," he said. "They've been on the air for three years."

The amount our lawyer worked so hard to get was $36,000.

Yet Jaime and I felt like the Beverly Hillbillies: *Load up the truck, Jethro, we're headin' to Hollywood!*

We just had absolutely no idea.

Then our trusty lawyer handed us two black Paper Mate pens.

"Well, here we go," I said as I wrote my name on the dotted line. "Signing our souls over to the devil."

Our lawyer laughed out loud.

It had been only a couple of months since the afternoon I'd rode the long escalator up to see Wendy in my white Dolce & Gabbana jacket and wings. I had no idea how far the angel was about to fall.

It was not until after I signed the contract that I told my mom about the show. Why would I tell her before? It was no surprise that she was very upset. "We are a private family," she said. "They're going to exploit us, our family name." She asked if we had control over editing (how savvy was Mom, huh?). "Yes, yes," I said, and I thought we did but we had no control, not even over the show's title. I remember our lawyer told us he pushed for that—Jaime and I had spent hours thinking of cool titles.

"What were you thinking?" my mother asked. "And what was your father thinking?"

I can't remember if I told her the title MTV had come up with. I probably didn't. It would have only agitated her more to know that her Alexandria was now the star of a reality television show called *Rich Girls*.

The night before we filmed the first episode I didn't sleep. I was shaky for some time before, as if my blood sugar was off. I kept eating PowerBars and protein shakes—I thought I must have been hypoglycemic, but doctors found only that I had low vitamin D levels and low iron. Later I found that all Lyme patients have extremely low vitamin D levels. All I knew is that I felt as though vibrating fire was running through my veins and to my head, and the only thing that would help was food. I had to have something in my purse to eat all the time so that I wouldn't feel lightheaded and woozy. I also didn't know at the time that not enough oxygen was making its way into my brain, a condition that I later learned is common in long-time Lyme sufferers.

Once the show started, there wasn't much time for me to just pop into a place to grab a quick bite. In order to do that, we would have to get filming clearance first and God forbid we went anywhere without the cameras. I stocked my purse full of lollipops so I could get the sugar when I needed it.

From the start, the show was a high-wire act without a net. There was no story line, plot, or even general direction toward a resolution. There weren't any plans for character development or setup for conflict (although plenty of that would organically arise). There were no good guys or bad guys (some of that would naturally happen, too). There was no structure. There was essentially nothing but Jaime and me, our so-called lives, and a rolling camera.

What could possibly go wrong?

The first show was about shopping for the prom. They rented a limo for us, a form of transportation that I would never use to just shop around New York. I usually just hop in a cab or, better yet, take the subway. We went to private showrooms with my "uncle" Michael H. Michael isn't really my uncle. Nonnie and Hippo sort of adopted him at an early age and he was best friends with Andy and Billy. As the camera followed, we spent ungodly amounts on our prom dresses (they zoomed in on the price tags). We had our hair done at Frederic Fekkai, a fancy midtown salon. We ate a late lunch in an Upper East Side restaurant. I was so tired during filming I couldn't think straight. I had full-on Lyme brain and didn't even know it.

I started to say things that I knew were incorrect but couldn't stop, like, "My dad invented cargo pants."

What? What the hell was I thinking?

I knew my dad didn't invent cargo pants; I was probably trying to say that he liked to design cargo pants. Too late. That one made it into the scene and ended up being one of the main things people like to make fun of me for saying.

After we wrapped ten or twelve hours of shooting, I couldn't help but think I'd made the biggest mistake doing the show and I had to shut up the voice of doom inside of me. I also felt trapped. Jaime was my best friend, and I didn't want to disappoint my best friend. I knew how much she wanted to be an actress. I knew she was wonderfully talented. I'm sure I told her how I felt, but I don't think I was forthright enough to make myself clear.

Meanwhile, my mom's voice was echoing in my head. As a teenager you don't want to do anything your mom says. Her little speech probably launched me into a mindset that said, "Yeah, fuck it. Now I'm really going to do it."

Looking back, I think maybe *Rich Girls* was the ultimate rebellion against my mom. I can see how screwed up my thinking was: *I'll show you: I'll hurt myself.*

eleven

WILFRED AND
THE BURRITO INCIDENT

*"If the disease [Lyme] remains untreated, a persistent
infection can occur after a few weeks or months, leading to
prolonged bouts of arthritis and neurologic problems, such as
concentration problems or personality changes."*
—NEW YORK TIMES

So you want to be a reality TV star? Well, consider this: For a ten-episode season, we shot six days a week, if not seven, ten to twelve hours a day, for five months. Jaime and I were miked all that time, constantly. The microphone consisted of a little cigarette pack-sized gizmo that you'd hook on to your skirt and then pull your shirt over, or hook to the back of your bra under your shirt. After you attach the gizmo, you thread a wire from up under your shirt and clip it or pin it to the inside of your collar. Then they put a little piece of tape on it to hold it there.

Pete, the soundman, was in his mid-forties and wore cargo shorts (which I don't think he invented) and had a reddish mustache. He looked as if he went hiking and rafting on the weekends and knew a lot about how to build a kick-ass campfire. He was the only one of the crew I really trusted because I believed he didn't have ulterior motives. Though we could ask Pete to turn off our mikes, like when we'd have to go to the bathroom, more times than not we'd forget that we were wearing them. Most of the day was so benign, so boring, that I'd even forget I was actually filming a television show that might be seen by a million people.

If you add up all the time that the cameras were rolling, the total comes to around 1,200 hours of audio and videotape—1,200 hours of tape whittled down to four hours of showtime. I'm not very good at fractions, but even I can figure out that with those numbers you can tell just about any story you want. I'm not saying I didn't give them material to work with; I did. Let's just say they were very good at editing.

In the beginning, I was a bit more in control of my actions in front of the camera. The first episode about shopping for the prom was pretty harmless and even charming in a way, and maybe even because of the few dumb things that came out of my mouth. What I didn't know at the time was that the Lyme disease was going to stage a full frontal assault. I didn't know that I was going to have a series of mini-breakdowns during the course of the five months of shooting. As those months wore on, nothing about the show felt harmless or charming. In fact, there were moments when I thought I would break emotionally right in front of the camera.

One Monday late in July, I had just come home from a quick and intense extended-family weekend trip to Nantucket. My dad's family has a lot of complicated dynamics. I'd just graduated from high school that June, and that weekend my family had asked a lot of questions: "What are you going to do now?" "Are you going to continue with the show? "How about working for your dad?"

I had to cut the trip short to come home to shoot, and when I woke up Monday morning I realized I had not planned anything for the show, which was my responsibility. The camera crew was on its way and I was alone in Dad's house. Shit. I might be witty when prompted by others, but alone, I just felt depressed and overwhelmed. I was also terribly hungover from the weekend.

For a fleeting moment, I had the idea that I'd paint for the camera. Painting was not only my greatest passion; it was my most comforting form of therapy. It was also an extremely personal activity. Back then, my ritual looked something like this: I would put on my painting clothes, usually sweatpants, an old graphic tee, and my Peggy Lipton beanie with all of my hair piled inside it. I would then put Crosby, Stills, Nash & Young's *Déjà vu* album on the stereo, roll the perfect joint, take a hit, and then gently tear open the plastic wrap of the canvas the same way a gentleman would seductively begin to make love to his lady. The canvas was my lover. If I'd painted on camera it would have been a huge betrayal of something I cared very deeply about.

Luckily, for the sake of my art I needed supplies and when I called the art store it was closed.

That left me without options for activities and I was too tired and Lyme-y to come up with anything else. Sitting around doing nothing is not compelling TV. I began to feel irresponsible. The crew had driven up from the city, people were getting paid, the director was pacing. Although they didn't say anything to me, I felt pressured to perform for them, or at least to try to think up something interesting for them to film me doing. Jaime had taken up the slack for me when I was away for the weekend, so it was my turn to be filmed alone so Jaime could have a little break.

My anxiety started to build, and filming began to spiral downward. I began to feel useless, not only as a reality television talent, but as a human being. I then asked myself the one question you really don't want to ask yourself on camera: *What am I going to do with my life?*

I guess I started to feel sorry for myself, but before I start beating myself up for sounding like a spoiled brat, let's face it: My childhood was screwed up. I'd grown up the eldest of four children and took the role of mother when my mother wasn't able to be there, which was for considerable amounts of time due to her strenuous hours working and going through bouts of emotional stress from the separation. My relationship with my mother was strained at this point, to say the least. She didn't understand what I was going through at all, which made me angry, and my anger turned into a deep sadness. My father leaned too much on me emotionally. I grew up way too fast, and without much parental guidance or supervision. In my teens, I was afforded absolutely no boundaries. It was as though my dad felt safer sharing his deepest feelings with me than he did with his wife. To this day, I believe his dependence on me in that way was a big strain on his relationship with my mom.

I, not my mom, accompanied my dad to all the affairs, dinners, and ceremonies. It was I who stood next to him against the step-and-repeat publicity backdrop while the cameras flashed. It was I who sat in the back of the limo or cab while he poured his heart out about business and deeply personal matters. I shouldn't have been a confidante, a peer—I should have been a daughter. I needed somebody to guide me and tell me what to do and what not to do. I needed direction and structure.

That day at my dad's, I started to feel out of control, scared, and so very lonely. I needed a container to hold what I was going through. My vessel was cracking, melting, crumbling, and I was desperate for somebody to provide the superglue to put it back together.

You should know that there's a deep loneliness to Lyme disease because nobody believes you about the pain and confusion. Your family, your friends, and even your doctors tell you it's all in your head, or that it's something else that's easily treatable. You feel like shit and they tell you you're beautiful, you're young, and you look fabulous. Wonderful! So you start to fool yourself. *Maybe they're right,* you say. *Maybe everybody feels just as shitty as I do.*

So when you go through fainting spells, you feel as if you're going to pass out or throw up, or you have extreme fatigue, joint pain, or crazy migraines, you make excuses up out of thin air: "I went running last week—that's why my knees hurt." "I have a headache because I'm dehydrated." As you pile the lies on top of each other, the distance between you and those close to you grows bigger and bigger until the day you realize you're in this ordeal all by yourself.

The confusion, physical pain, and heart palpitations Lyme disease causes are torment enough. Add a hangover, a camera crew for a reality TV show, loneliness, and, well, what you get is just what happened to me: I started to break down.

And I could think of only one person to talk to about it.

On the phone with Dad that day I was a lost little girl as the cameras rolled. Although I haven't seen the episode in many years, remembering now how I exposed myself so publicly still makes me cringe. I came across like the spoiled brat I warned you about, whining and crying about how hard my life was while I was walking around Dad's swimming pool. This was the first time I got really personal and private on camera. It was actually funny that my attempt at getting deeply personal with kids in New York was my goal, yet I was totally unwilling to reveal what was going on behind closed doors in my own personal life. I think part of me was taking some of my mother's moral upbringing when it came to privacy, which is even funnier, because filming a reality television show is the *exact* opposite of being private.

It was my worst nightmare, and the polar opposite of what I had hoped the show would be.

I remember feeling scared and lonely and desperate to figure out what I was going to do with my life, something that had meaning. The life I had created with cameras following me around was not the life I intended to lead. I wanted to turn back time and erase what I had done. I wanted to go back into my childhood, before everything became so hard.

As I poured my heart out to my dad I forgot the cameras. I didn't think about how I would look on television crying about my life, to families torn apart in much worse ways than mine, to children who had no family to speak of, or to single mothers trying to make ends meet. My life seemed and was pretty damn great compared to most. In a way I suppose I achieved that day, in a small way, what I actually wanted the show to be about: No matter how much you have, how you grow up, where you live, how tall you are, or what skin color you have, we all have issues and life to sort through.

Obviously mine were petty issues next to racial profiling and murder, but they were symbolic of a daily struggle everyone goes though. Unfortunately, the editing team at MTV didn't get that the audience may have related to my honest emotions. Nope. They just saw it as a great big opportunity to make fun of a teenage girl going through one of life's biggest transitions: teenagehood to real adulthood. Actually, what they were seeing was a girl having a Lyme breakdown and starting to shut down.

* * *

After the phone call to my dad, the episode devolved into theater of the absurd. I decided that the only thing that could help me was a burrito. There was nothing in my dad's refrigerator, and I wasn't about to order in food and wait for an hour and a half, sitting around being nervous or just flat-out fainting on camera. I thought it would make for an interesting on-camera activity for me to go to the grocery store and buy the ingredients to make burritos.

Now, picture walking into a small grocery store on a summer holiday, and then picture walking in with a camera crew of four. *Seriously? I am actually doing this? No one will let me go anywhere ever again!* I also had no idea what kind of specific ingredients went into making a burrito. All I knew was that I needed something to eat and that I had better make something fast or I might pass out. Or maybe my head would just spin right off. That would have made for an interesting episode.

Once I managed to buy all the ingredients, I walked out to the parking lot with all of my bags in hand, the camera crew in tow, and I stopped to chat with the parking lot attendant. This man was a gentle soul, a man I knew had been through a lot in his life. He was real. He was authentic and grounded. He was what I wanted to be, who I needed to be around.

"How are you today, Wilfred?"

"I'm fine, miss. How are you doing on this sunny day?"

"Well, I am okay. I am going home to make some burritos. . . ."

In the back of my mind I was secretly asking him to kidnap me, take me home with him to his little family, where I could live a simple and normal life.

I gazed into his tired, watery eyes for much longer than I should have, wondering if he could read my mind, if he could understand the agony that I was putting myself through. I wondered if he knew I was different from the other women who drove through his parking lot, impatient and hushing their spoiled, crying children in the backseats of their Mercedes station wagons. I didn't know why I was making the choices I was making and didn't have a clue that at least some of my craziness was not my fault at all.

I arrived home and called one of my closest friends at the time, Danielle. I needed someone else on camera with me and to help me make the burritos. All I wanted was to eat as soon as possible, and in a comfortable environment. My heart had been racing the whole day, my hands felt shaky, and I couldn't think clearly anymore. Partly this was because of the hangover. But it was also a feeling I often had without having a hangover at all. I didn't know this then, but Lyme sufferers can feel as though they have a hangover every single day, whether or not they take a single drink. What makes it even more diabolical is you don't look like absolute death; you just feel that way.

As soon as Danielle came to the house, I hugged her and immediately began to chop onions. Danielle knew how to make rice, and I knew how to chop onions. We didn't know how to cook or season ground beef or how to cook beans.

Danielle began asking me questions. "What do you want to do while the rice is cooking? What kind of seasoning should we put on the beef? Do you need the beans? What about lettuce? Did you know that burritos have a lot of carbs? What do you want to do after we eat? Where do you want to eat? How did the earth come to exist? Why do you think toenails are the shape and color they are? How do I break up with my boyfriend? What are you going to do after the summer? Do you think your parents will ever get back together?

What do you want me to help you with? Ally, Ally? Ally? Are you okay . . . ?"

Brain shutting down. Come back to life, Ally. Come on, make words come out of your mouth.

"Danielle, I am starving. All I want is to have the rice, with beef, on a plate, and in my mouth, as soon as humanly possible. I feel like I do not know how to make a decision as simple as how much salt I need to shake into the pan right now."

"Well, we have a lot of options. We could not eat, eat, order in, sit outside, go upstairs, take a nap. . . . What do you feel like doing?"

I grabbed Danielle's hand and ran outside and we jumped into the swimming pool with all of our clothes on—microphones still attached. I dragged her with me. I didn't care what happened. I wanted to escape and feel free, and it was the only way to shut her up. It looked like a fun, innocent, and lighthearted thing to do in the moment, but little did anyone know, I was so overwhelmed that all I could do was jump into deep cold water to numb out.

I knew alcohol wasn't the answer. I knew I had drunk enough that weekend, and I didn't want to be totally annihilated on-screen. And all I wanted to do was eat a fucking burrito.

At some point during the filming I just started to barrel through. I wanted to get the show over with. I will admit that I wasn't at my best—not by a mile. I was smoking pot just about every night because of my achy joints and the need to escape the harsh reality of making reality TV.

When my friend Liz Meyer joined *Rich Girls,* things really became unhinged. Jaime and Liz didn't get along. It was almost as though they were competing for my friendship. I know that sounds terribly self-centered, but that's how it seemed to me. The conflict was actually highlighted in the show.

The discomfort of the situation pervaded every part of my life. The show used a lot of interviews where I was alone and talked right to the camera, a format that is now a reality TV staple. The reason they're a staple is that there is so much pressure on the person being interviewed—the viewer doesn't see the camera, the lights, and the crew. But I was defensive and, most of the time, brutally honest.

One time when we were shooting interviews in a hotel, I was exhausted, so drained. The show wasn't supposed to create rifts in my relationships. I was fed up with both Jaime and Liz and their childish behavior, and pissed at them because they had put me in this awkward situation. The director was asking me really uncomfortable questions about my friendships and perspectives on Jaime and Liz, questions that I did not feel comfortable answering, because I didn't want to hurt either of their feelings. Then, in the middle of the interview, I told the crew to turn off the cameras and I walked into a bathroom. I crawled onto the bath mat and began to sob. I felt so trapped, so freaked out, that I just wanted to end my life. The show hadn't even aired yet and it was killing me.

I was going a million miles an hour, there was so much scheduling, securing releases from restaurants, hotels, and stores. We were constantly trying to come up with ideas for the show. It was like living a double life in the fast lane.

By the end of summer, we had already been filming for four and a half months and I was not feeling well. I was nauseous most of the time, and my knees and hips were killing me. Sleeping was becoming increasingly difficult, too, which didn't help me feel awake and chipper during the day. I remember being aware of how slowly I was speaking from the fatigue. I think it came across on camera as if I was smoking my weed during the day, rather than in the evening. We had planned to shoot a trip to Seattle and I remember telling my mom I didn't want to go.

"Well, honey," she said, "then don't."

Oh, how I wanted to just take a bath, get into my mom's pretty sheets, curl up in front of the fire, drink chamomile tea, and watch old movies or *I Love Lucy*. I needed to feel that nostalgia, the warmth. I needed my mommy.

twelve

TURNING TO JUDAISM IN A KARAOKE NIGHTCLUB

"Rarely, patients with undetected Lyme disease may present with obsessive compulsive disorder, paranoia, auditory/visual hallucinations, or full blown mania."
—COLUMBIA UNIVERSITY MEDICAL CENTER

The first week after the show wrapped is a blur. I remember I painted my head off, which means I smoked a lot of weed, locked myself in my art studio, and experimented on the canvas for hours on end. I went into the city to my dad's office a few times a week to help him with his collections. I liked to help my dad at work, and he appreciated my opinions.

Hanging out with my dad after the season wrapped was perfect because it took my mind off *Rich Girls* and the internal criticism that played on a loop in my thoughts. I went on a business trip with him and his team to attend some press junkets and do some sample shopping. In this kind of shopping you're looking for inspiration. You travel to stores throughout Europe searching for fabrics, colors, or patterns that kindle your imagination. It's one of the most enjoy-

able aspects of designing for a large corporation. I was not technically an employee, but I was a part of the team, and I was the most
enthusiastic of the whole group.

Now that the show was over, I felt as if I'd been let out of jail or
saved from a sinking ship. I felt as if I were the luckiest person on
earth to be on a sample shopping trip through Europe. We went to
Berlin, Amsterdam, and Paris. A lot of the trip, however, is lost in
my memory.

When we got back to the States at the end of September, and after
attending the show's premier party in Los Angeles (where I did *The
Sharon Osbourne Show*), we had a launch party in New York. I went
to the party with my friend Charlie. I knew Charlie from a guy I was
dating, and he had been my most awesome best friend. Charlie did
something very unexpected: He kissed me. I was totally shocked. I
hadn't thought of him in a sexual way at all.

I don't know how much the kiss had to do with it, but soon after
the party I decided to go to Miami to visit Charlie. He was attending the University of Miami at the time and sharing a bungalow in
South Beach with a couple of friends. As soon as I arrived, I knew I
didn't want to leave. We were near the ocean, and smell of the sea air
and the feel of the sand between my toes reminded me of Mustique.
I felt as if I had escaped into a secret special world where I could play
house and act like a big kid. With Charlie and his friends I had a
blast. We played basketball or went to the beach during the day. At
night we'd sing karaoke at a cheesy joint owned by an ex–Garment
District guy named Marty, who told me, "I sold mannequins to your
father in the eighties."

Either I started to see Charlie in a more romantic light or I just
felt safe and comfortable with him, and I began to think I could

marry him and live in Miami forever. I thought I might audit classes at the University of Miami and make a home.

I found something comfortable also about being around people of the Jewish faith. Charlie is Jewish, and his friends Andrew and Stephen are very dedicated to the Jewish faith. I loved the importance that laughter and warmth played in the families of the Jewish people I've known. On Mayfair Lane our neighbors and friends were the Coguts. They would invite us over for Seder dinner. I loved it: It was formal but friendly and so deep and full of meaning. I was only a little girl, but I understood the importance of the ritual.

I sat next to Ga Ga, one of the Cogut grandmothers and a Holocaust survivor, and had the most incredible conversations with her. I wasn't afraid to ask her questions about her life, and she wasn't afraid to answer them. There were tears, laughter, and hugs and in those talks. I felt wonderfully warm with them.

A lot of my father's business sense came from his Jewish partners' way of thinking, and that sense was passed down to me. I adored my father's business partners Lawrence Stroll, who had the biggest heart; Joel Horowitz, who was a mensch and very funny; and Silas Chou, who though was not Jewish was a wise and witty Chinese man I considered to be the neck—the strength—of the whole brand. They were our family.

I felt the same way with Charlie. So I started studying the Torah and looking into the process of converting to Judaism. When I told my mother I was thinking of converting she said, "I wish there was a Jewish pill I could give all my children to make them instantly Jewish."

Truth was, I needed a good friend and shoulder to cry on much more than a lover or a husband. That was why I clung to Charlie so tightly.

When the MTV show aired in October, a bunch of us Miami friends gathered in Charlie's living room. We laughed and hollered and made fun of the show from head to toe. Though it felt good to laugh at myself, and I was impressed at the clever way they edited us to make us look a lot more ridiculous than we actually were (I had to admit, it kept the show interesting and engaging), I began to feel a little embarrassed that I was on national television acting like a dumb rich girl.

Had I been in another place physically and emotionally, I might have given myself credit for a producing a show that was on the front end of a television phenomenon that would dominate the television entertainment world. But I wasn't in that place, so instead I kept sneaking off to the refrigerator to take little nips out of a Jäger bottle to round off the edges of anxiety I was feeling.

There were a couple of redeeming moments during *Rich Girls*. We filmed Bill Clinton awarding commendation medals, forty years overdue, to the surviving sailors from the USS *Mason*. The ceremony took place on the deck of the new USS *Mason*, named after the original and docked that day in New York Harbor. We also filmed my class's graduation from PCS, an event in which I was awarded high honors.

At some point I received a call from Wendy at MTV telling me that the show was getting some of the highest ratings numbers they had seen in a while, but what she said was lost on me. Though intellectually I knew what it meant, on a deep emotional level I couldn't process the information. I just wanted it all to go away, so I talked myself into the idea that the show was a bust. I began to realize otherwise one day at a gas station in Miami. Charlie waited for me in the car as I ran in to buy a pack of gum. In the store, I thought people were staring at me but I shrugged it off as paranoia until someone asked if they could take a photo of me. If I didn't know then that my life had changed, I found out for sure a couple of days later.

Besides playing basketball or tennis at Andrew's and going to Marty's for karaoke at night, I didn't go out much in Miami. Charlie ran most of the errands. One day, however, I decided to go to the Target store in Coral Gables to do some shopping. I always like the big, red shopping carts they have in Target—they make me feel like I'm a kid again.

So off I went. I don't even think I'd brushed my teeth that morning. I had my hair in dreadlocks with massive red string wrapped in them. I was feeling shitty physically. The nausea, which had started during filming of the show, had been growing worse and I felt as if my heart were beating out of my chest. (I didn't know then that heart palpitations are a common symptom in Lyme sufferers.) I couldn't walk very well due to swollen joints, and my memory was becoming weaker.

I'd gone to Target to buy lanterns and other lights for Charlie's garden but there were so many twinkle lights to choose from, I started to get a headache. Normal people take a short amount of time to make simple decisions, but you would have thought I was deciding on my wedding dress. Decision making had become so challenging for me that often I would just close my eyes, point, and click, so to speak.

Anyway, I was standing there staring at the lights for I don't know how long when I had the sensation of people looking at me. I turned around and a group of about six shoppers was watching me. "You're Ally from *Rich Girls*," one of them said in an amazed way. A woman aimed her flip-phone at me to take a photo. I felt like an animal in a zoo. "What are you doing in Coral Gables?" another asked. "What are you doing in Target!" a woman squealed.

My anxious answers became long-winded and scattered. I decided to zip it when I realized that I was divulging unnecessary amounts of personal information. I signed autographs and posed for pictures, but I couldn't wait to get away. I couldn't imagine how people with enduring fame handled this.

I began to full-on freak out when the same scenario repeated itself several more times in the store. I paid for the lanterns and then barreled out, pushing the basket in front of me. I remember thinking, *Oh, my God. I can never go to a store again.*

Though my time in Miami was mostly fun and had its moments of normalcy, I was living in a state of compete denial about *Rich Girls*. While I was floating around in this state of denial, a part of my soul had broken off and was now on people's television sets and making me a celebrity. It was such a strange time in my life—as if I existed between two worlds. For a time I was able to manage it. But in moments like the one at Target, when the my two worlds collided, I was left with a question that shook me to my core.

How do I live the rest of my life?

thirteen

FROM THE ER TO BUNGALOW 8

"Lyme carditis occurs when Lyme disease bacteria enter the tissues of the heart. This can interfere with the normal movement of electrical signals from the heart's upper to lower chambers, a process that coordinates the beating of the heart. The result is something physicians call 'heart block,' which can be mild, moderate, or severe. Heart block from Lyme carditis can progress rapidly."
—CENTERS FOR DISEASE CONTROL AND PREVENTION

Despite my denial, *Rich Girls* was a breakout hit, exceeding even the most optimistic predictions. Everyone, it seemed, was talking about it. That Thanksgiving, my father wanted the family to gather on Mustique. We rented out two houses on the island to hold the overflow of cousins, uncles, and aunts. When everyone gets together it is chaotic, fun, crazy, and unpredictable. Complicated. Still, I'm usually excited to spend time with them. On this trip, however, I had an enormous amount of emotional baggage. I was worried sick about the family's reaction to the show and did whatever I could to not talk about it.

When I got back to Miami I began to experience more severe bouts of nausea. During one attack, Charlie took me to the emergency room. The doctor asked about my medical history. I told him I had been diagnosed with rheumatoid arthritis, multiple sclerosis, and fibromyalgia, which I'd been treated for, and that I had suffered through major panic attacks in the recent years. I told him about my ovarian cysts, which had sent me to the hospital twice, causing the doctors to prescribe me birth control pills to dissolve the cysts. The damn pills made me so nauseous and depressed from the weight gain and water retention that I stopped taking them two years prior to living in Miami. I told him that, despite all of the treatments I'd been on and all the doctors I'd seen, no one could really tell me what was wrong with me.

In the ER they couldn't, either. I wasn't pregnant, I didn't have appendicitis, and the blood work they took came back normal (I think). They put a catheter in me at one point, God knows why, but it had me screaming in agony. They found that I had a permanent heart murmur but said it was nothing serious.

No one could figure out what was going on.

Afterward I felt well enough to take a trip to Orlando to visit my cousin Jaimie. On the way back, however, I couldn't get on the plane because I was paranoid. I thought people were following me. I thought someone was going to blow up the plane. I thought I was being watched.

I started to think about Jaime and *Rich Girls*. I'd refused to do any talk shows or interviews, and I knew she was mad at me. I also knew I couldn't even think of the show, let alone talk about it, without experiencing severe anxiety. My panic at the airport led to an attack of nausea. It hit me right as I was going through security. Every few minutes I had to run to a garbage can to vomit.

A tall, black man with a shiny security badge, weathered face, kind eyes, and big hands took me to a room so I could calm down and call my father. My dad basically told me to just try to relax and get on the flight. He didn't understand that I was really starting to unravel. The security man reminded me of Wilfred from the burrito episode. He bought me a Coca-Cola, and told me to take small sips and to put salt on the end of my tongue to help stop the nausea. He sat with me and I cried in his arms. I wanted to go home with him and eat his wife's meat loaf or something. All I really wanted was a simple home life.

I decided I would just drive home to Miami. I took the shuttle to the car rental and waited in line. I'd never rented a car before and didn't know I had to be twenty-five. When they told me I couldn't take a car, I had another mini-breakdown and cried. I wandered across the street to a beautiful lawn with a beautiful little tree, which I climbed and sat in for about four hours. I sang little songs to myself and wrote poetry. Maybe I could just stay in the tree, I thought. Finally, I called Charlie and he drove all the way to Orlando to rescue me.

The next day I was in the Miami hospital again, this time with headaches along with the severe nausea. When they took my blood pressure, it was out of whack. After I was released, I checked into the Shore Club hotel in Miami, where I stayed for a couple of weeks—I didn't want to be sick in front of Charlie's friends. At the Shore Club, I was assigned bungalow number 8 on the beach, which made me smile. Bungalow 8 was then a popular nightclub in Manhattan, but I was very far from clubbing mode. I was living on Pedialyte, saltine crackers, and Marlboro Lights. I was also taking the occasional hit off a joint to sooth the waves of nausea. Just the thought of alcohol made my stomach heave. I kept my father in the loop about what was going on and at one point he flew down to check on me. He spoke to me mostly about what I was going to do next with my future. This only added to the anxiety and nausea.

At some point Charlie's friend Andrew called his brother, who was a doctor. The doctor and his wife came to visit me at the Shore Club. It was the doctor's wife who saw what was wrong: "Honey," she said, "your nausea is coming from tremendous amounts of anxiety."

I knew she was right. In that moment I knew it was the show that was making me even sicker that I'd already been before. I knew I had to cut it out of my life like a cancer or I would never get better.

If I had any doubt about what I should do, Charlie put it to rest. He had stayed with me through many of these hospital visits and took great care of me. He witnessed the anxiety and paranoia I experienced when people recognized me. He knew the show wasn't good for me and the strain I was feeling in my relationship with Jaime.

My costar and I had grown very distant, and I was afraid to tell her that I didn't want to do the talk shows, TV spots, or magazine interviews, let alone film a second season. I had distanced myself from her because I thought she probably enjoyed filming and the glow of the spotlight, whereas I was turned off by it. I felt violated by it.

What I didn't know was that Lyme disease was causing me so much pain and mental disorder that it was impossible for me to do what the show and Jaime wanted.

Charlie gave me an ultimatum. He told me that he couldn't be with me anymore if I didn't call Jaime and tell her that I could no longer be part of the show. Charlie had stayed through the darkest part of my life. His only agenda was caring for me. I picked up my phone and I dialed Jaime.

On the phone I was cold, emotionless. I think I left my body a little bit. I just told her the truth but did so in a rude and blunt way. I wasn't going to have any part in the show anymore, I said. I didn't care about the contract—I would get out of it somehow. I told her that I no longer wanted to be her friend.

I didn't show an ounce of compassion or remorse. I just ripped off the Band-Aid as rapidly as I could. I wanted the nausea to stop once and for all and I believed in my heart that cutting my ties to Jaime and *Rich Girls* was the only way that would happen.

Now I feel bad about how I handled the situation, but when I hung up the phone that day I felt as though a great weight had lifted off my shoulders. For the first time in weeks I didn't feel nauseous at all. I thought Charlie and the doctor's wife were right: It was the anxiety over *Rich Girls* that made me sick to my stomach.

A few days after I called Jaime, I flew back to New York. It was mid-December and I wanted to be with my family for Christmas. I really thought everything was going to be better.

Nothing could have been further from the truth.

fourteen

COMMENCING COUNTDOWN, ENGINES ON...

"Disruptions caused by GI borreliosis [Lyme] may include, amongst many others, distortions of taste, failure of other neural functions that supply the entire GI tract—paralysis or partial paralysis of the tongue, gag reflex, esophagus, stomach and nearby organs. . . ."
—VIRGINIA T. SHERR, M.D.

The last two weeks of December 2003 form in my memory like a series of Polaroid snapshots.

The first one that comes into focus is perhaps the most random. After I landed in New York City, I went to a middle school in Harlem where my uncle Andy and cousin Mike Fredo were performing in a Christmas pageant. They asked me to come and sing along with them. I felt safe and normal with Andy and Mike, and singing in the Harlem middle school was as far away from *Rich Girls* as I could get.

Except, as it turned out, people in Harlem watched *Rich Girls*, too, and several of the kids asked about the show. I felt none of the anxiety, however, that I'd had in Florida. It was fun. I kept it low-key and deflected the attention. For a moment, it was as though I had truly left the worst behind and a new life beckoned.

The next scene I remember is being with my friend Danielle driving to Chelsea Piers in Manhattan to go bowling with some of her college guy friends. But instead of bowling we went to a hamburger place nearby called Lucky's. Don't ask me why, but for some reason I was able to eat Lucky's hamburgers without getting nauseous. Remember, I was on a straight diet of Pedialyte up until then. I had no inclination to drink alcohol, but I was still medicating myself with weed. It really did help with my stomach. Maybe it had something to do with Lucky's hamburgers tasting so good.

I was drinking a lot of water, maybe three or four liters a day. I felt as if I was almost getting high off the water. I felt so dehydrated, and I had a strong instinct that I just needed to flush and hydrate.

I'd parked my car, a navy blue 2001 Range Rover with tan interior, in a covered lot at Chelsea Piers. The Range Rover became my home. I called people, like my cousin Jennifer, to come visit me there. "We'll get burgers!" I'd exclaim. It was almost as though I'd made the decision to live out of my car, and I did for a week, maybe two. I didn't sleep in my car, but I'd spend a lot of time just sitting inside it because I felt safe and somewhat anonymous.

Though it sounds strange recounting this period of my life, back then it didn't seem strange at all!

I don't know how much I slept during that time. I think I went to my mom's house and hung out with her one night and maybe walked across the street to my dad's. I vaguely remember driving up to Danielle's college in Massachusetts and staying there for a couple of sleepless nights.

It dawned on me at one point that I should probably go Christmas shopping. Then I really started going crazy. When buying gifts for family and friends, I had no sense of reality, no sense of how much money one should or shouldn't spend. I drove up to Connecticut and visited a jewelry store to go random gift shopping. I saw this beautiful, 1920s headband, something a flapper would wear, and I bought it for myself for Christmas. (I might have been going crazy, but my sense of style was intact. I still wear the piece. It's beautiful.)

The jeweler was in the back of the store when I first saw him, working on the jewelry, but then he came out front to help with customers. I took one look at him and for a reason I still cannot fully explain I said, "Hey, you have to tell your sons that you and your wife are separating."

The look of shock on the poor man's face is still clear in my memory. He was middle-aged, Jewish. "Do I know you?" he asked. I think I shrugged. "How do you know these things?" he insisted. I must have opened up psychically, because I'd nailed him. He told me that he and his wife were discussing divorce and that he did have a couple of sons he hadn't told yet. I walked out of the store with my newly purchased 1920s era headband, content that I'd helped the man. (I don't think I helped him at all, actually; I think I just totally freaked him out. The whole episode was something out of *The Twilight Zone*.)

The next scene I remember is crying on the floor of a bathroom in my father's house. I'd hit a wall with my physical ailments. I couldn't think straight. I was overwhelmed and confused. I couldn't figure out how to do the simplest things, like make a phone call, take a shower, or make myself something to eat—let alone try to organize Christmas gifts for my friends and family. For fucksake, I didn't even know how to go to sleep. And all I wanted was to go to sleep. I felt as if I was falling apart.

My dad came into the huge bathroom. I'd been complaining about hurting and not feeling well for a long, long time. I hadn't had an outburst in a while but I could feel one welling up in me like lava in a little volcano. He kept asking, "Ally, please, what can I do to help you, honey? Can I run you a bath? Get you a massage? Make you some food? Just tell me what I can do to help you."

"Those things don't work," I said. "Call and get me some weed. The only thing that works is weed."

I think it was then that my dad started to believe that I was a major drug addict, which only made me more furious.

"You just don't listen!" I screamed.

I then had a brilliant idea. Back in high school, post 9/11, I'd gone to see a healer and recorded all my sessions with her. I still had the recordings. I walked out of the bathroom and put the audiotape from my healing sessions into the sound system of my dad's house and turned the volume way up so he could hear them. This way he would believe that I really was sick and not addicted to drugs. I thought if he heard it from the healer's mouth he would believe me.

I didn't know I had Lyme disease, I was just searching for some cause for how bad I felt. I knew multiple sclerosis and fibromyalgia were not the correct diagnoses. I don't know how I knew, but I just did. There were too many missing pieces and too little clarity around the blood tests and treatments. Some of my family members had come back from the Thanksgiving weekend in Mustique with parasites. It certainly would have made sense that I'd had one, considering how I felt. I kept saying, "There are bugs in me, there's something foreign living inside of me." I felt as though my stomach were eating itself all the time. I would eat a plate of food and feel as if I had eaten absolutely nothing, another typical result of Lyme disease.

With the healer's voice still echoing through my father's house, I left and went over to my mom's house across the street. In the midst of this insanity, I was still experiencing some kind of psychic breakthrough. I called some of my friends in Greenwich and invited them to my mom's. I remember talking a mile a minute to them on the phone. I was so anxious to tell them about the revelations I was having.

If you asked me today what those revelations were, I don't think I'd be able to tell you. I do remember the basic theme of them, however—truth. I remember it being of absolute and paramount importance that a person accept the truth of who she is and not hide behind any façade.

At one point I felt like I was channeling Bob Marley and speaking in a singsong Rasta accent. I really didn't know anything about Bob Marley, except for a few of his popular songs, but suddenly I thought I did. I was also carrying around spiritual books—the one by Mother Teresa and *The Power of Now,* which my mother had given me over the years—and pine needles in my pocket. I'd rub and inhale them—the scent seemed to help my nausea.

I thought fans from the television show were trying to get to me in my mother's house. The only people I really trusted were her security guards. They were regular guys who didn't buy into all the materialism bullshit. I didn't go anywhere without them. Even when I had to go to the bathroom I'd ask one of them to stand outside the door. I still couldn't sleep, so they'd stay up all night with me. In the middle of the night, when everyone was asleep in my mother's house, I'd sit in the living room with the guards, smoking cigarettes and reading Tarot for them. I didn't have real Tarot cards, so I used a regular deck of cards. It wouldn't have mattered if I were reading bar coasters. The clarity I had into their lives astounds me still.

You must know I am not claiming to be some incredible psychic. It's scary to share the truth of what happened to me during that time. I can't understand why and what happened exactly, but I do know that it sure as hell happened. At the time, what came out my mind and mouth were so uncontrollable, and I didn't have time to process or slow down what was going on. I was flooded with these thoughts and insights and I wasn't making sense half the time. I was not in my right mind enough even to scare myself with the way I was behaving.

In the next scene, on Christmas Eve, I decided I needed to go into New York City. I knew I wouldn't be able to drive because the task just seemed so overwhelming, so I talked my mother's boyfriend and one of her assistants into driving me.

In the car, I called just about everyone I'd known for a length of time who lived in New York. Most of them didn't pick up; the ones who did asked why I wasn't home with my family like they were on Christmas Eve.

It was on this drive that I ended up in the church. I made my mother's boyfriend stop at St. Patrick's, the Catholic church in Bedford Village, New York, where we used to go. I remember that I was wearing a Marc Jacobs blood-orange mod coat, flared Levi jeans, and red, orange, and navy blue Adidas sneakers, with my hair in two huge dreads, and still carrying the Mother Teresa book in my hand and the pine needles in my pocket. When I was a child, I loved the smell of Christmas trees; maybe the pine needles also reminded me of a time when everything in my life felt safe and good. Now I was standing in the middle of Midnight Mass, which should have been called Midnight Madness in my case, feeling as if I was losing my mind.

A family I knew from Greenwich was there. I knew they had suffered a loss of family member not too long before, so I gave them the Mother Teresa book. I stayed in St. Patrick's until the church had cleared. I thought that maybe the priest could help me go to sleep. When I was thirteen I'd refused to receive the sacrament of confirmation because I'd decided that I did not believe in the Catholic religion. Here I was on Christmas Eve falling to my knees and weeping in front of a priest. I felt as though he was my last resort, and I begged him to help me.

He put his hand over my head and said something like, "Lord Jesus Christ, help bestow sleep upon this child tonight." Then my mother's boyfriend drove me to my father's house, where I passed out and slept for about fourteen hours.

I remember very little about Christmas Day. Charlie's friends from Miami, Andrew and Stephen, were with me, because I felt safe with them. I vaguely recall making them stay with me as I tried to sleep and telling them that I felt like there were bugs inside my body.

The next day I do remember.

I was in my mom's house painting when my dad came into the room. "Ally, I think you have to go to Silver Hill," he said.

"The rehab? The psych ward?" I said.

"The other day when you told me that the only thing that can help you is weed, that scared me."

Then I threw whatever I could get my hands on across the room and smashed a huge dresser mirror. As my father turned to leave, I yelled, "You don't know what you're talking about and you're not listening to me! That's not what's wrong with me! You're the crazy one!"

My mom didn't think I needed to go to rehab; she thought I needed to see a psychic. The next thing I knew I was sitting across from a psychic who was telling me how specially gifted I was. I really didn't want to hear anything she had to say.

That day my dad flew to Colorado for a planned trip and I had one of my mom's security guards drive me into the city again, this time so I could find Ms. Sclan, my English teacher from PCS. I thought she would understand what I was going through. I couldn't find Ms. Sclan's number. I knew she liked to eat at Steak Frites near Union Square, but for some reason we didn't go there and instead settled for a bar on MacDougal Street in Greenwich Village.

I felt like shit. My father wanted me to go to rehab. *I might as well just get drunk,* I thought. The place was called Off the Wagon. Pretty appropriate, huh?

At the bar that night, I told the security guard my deepest secrets. I hadn't even told my parents, but here I was pouring my heart out to the security guard. I was desperate for anyone's compassion; maybe someone would be able to explain what the hell was happening to me.

Later my dad told me that I called him that night and asked for help in a way that frightened him. My dad was still in Colorado. It was the middle of the night and snowing heavily there, but my dad decided to fly home anyway. He remembers getting into a taxi and the driver seeming a little sketchy. Dad must have looked pretty worried. He feared for his daughter's life, the snow was coming sideways, he didn't know if the plane would take off, and he didn't really trust the guy who was driving him to the airport. But then the driver turned to my dad and asked him if he was okay.

"No," my dad said. And he told the guy behind the wheel the whole story. As it happened, the driver was the perfect audience. He'd had problems with his daughter, too, but she was sober for ninety days now. The driver himself had been sober for many years. My dad took this as a sign that his daughter needed to go to rehab.

I woke up late the next afternoon to find my father waiting for me in the kitchen. I was still very angry at him. I kept telling him that I was sick, that something was wrong inside me. I began to think about the parasites again and that he wasn't getting the message. I got out of bed, grabbed a silver tray off a table, went into the bathroom, defecated on it, and handed it to him.

"You've gotta get this tested," I said. "If there are parasites in there you're going to be sorry."

In looking back, I can't blame him or anyone else for thinking that I was off my rocker. Even in my crazy manic state, however, I knew there was something physically wrong with me and that no matter how hard I screamed, no one heard. The louder I screamed, the less they listened, and the more they thought I was nuts.

I remember standing in the foyer in my mother's house, in my underwear, weighing about eighty-seven pounds and using a wooden spoon to smash my mother's favorite plates, acting like George in *Who's Afraid of Virginia Woolf?* One of my mom's security guards had a sister or girlfriend who was a therapist, and my father had called her so she was in the house while I was smashing the plates. Everybody was trying to reason with me, but it was as if we were speaking different languages: I was yelling, "Help me!" And they were saying, "It's okay."

I don't know whether it was because of my sudden Bob Marley obsession, but I decided I had to go to Jamaica. The answer to my problems, I thought, must be in Jamaica. At the time, my mom's assistant, Isa, who happens to be Michael Bolton's daughter, was in Jamaica with her family on a Christmas vacation, so I thought I would go visit them.

Finally it seemed my dad heard what I was trying to say. "Okay," he said. "I'll take you to the airport and we'll go to Jamaica." I went upstairs, took a shower, and put some stuff into a suitcase. When I came downstairs, my dad grabbed me and shoved pills down my throat. He was hurting me and I looked toward the security guard for help. He said, "Mr. Hilfiger, take your hands off your daughter," and my dad released me but the pills had already dissolved. They did calm me down.

They took me to out to the car while my mother screamed, "Do not take her! Do not take her!" Her boyfriend was holding her back, but Mom was kicking and screaming. She was trying to help me but she didn't know how. They put me in the backseat with a security guard on either side and my dad drove.

It soon became apparent that we were not headed toward the airport. "Where are you taking me?" I asked.

"Ally, I'm taking you to the emergency room."

I yelled at Dad to let me out. I was afraid there would be cameras and reporters and people would recognize me at the hospital. One of the guards assured me that we were going in a back entrance, that it was private and no one would know. Inside the hospital door, a doctor was waiting for us. The thought of seeing a doctor calmed me down enough that I walked into the emergency room without a struggle.

And that's when I started playing with a purple glove while he injected me with something . . . and *blackout*.

part two

fifteen

ONE FLEW OVER THE CUCKOO'S NEST

"I must be crazy to be in a loony bin like this."
—RANDALL PATRICK MCMURPHY

I personally believe that most things happen for a reason, and that our instincts guide us toward those who are divinely meant to be in our lives. I also believe that we have had many lives before this one, and that we make "soul agreements" with other people before entering into the next life. I know this theory might sound totally out there, but it's a belief that I've deeply explored, questioned, and proved in mysterious ways throughout the years. There are wonderful books on the subject that explain it a lot better than I can.

Throughout my life I've found kindred spirits in people much older than I am. I think of them as spiritual guides who are placed in my path, one after another, literally handing me along.

Some of this conviction comes from my dad's Hindu beliefs, although my father leans more toward the Buddhist teachings. I've mentioned that in the early days, my parents traveled to India often to make their clothes. They lived there for a while right after they were married, when dad was making 20th Century Survival and mom had O Tokyo. Mohan Murjani, who backed my father in business, is a Hindu Indian. Mohan gave us a prayer book called *Begin the Day with God* and every evening at dinner my mom would choose one of us to read out of the book. Later, I'd devoured books like *Teachings of the Buddha,* by Jack Kornfield; *Your Soul's Plan,* by Robert Schwartz; *Many Lives, Many Masters,* by Brian L. Weiss, M.D.; and *The Alchemist,* by Paulo Coelho. It was these readings and other sources that introduced me to the idea of past lives.

If I had any flicker of doubt about living past lives, it was extinguished by the connection I've had with my dad. Over the years we've had too many moments of déjà vu, too much intuition and unexplained affinity for the same things to doubt that we have been here together before.

So it was very difficult for me to accept that my father had committed me to a psychiatric hospital. I thought he'd done it because of some past-life debits that I owed, perhaps to him. I realize this sounds nuts, but sometimes your best insights come when you're at your most messed up. Think about that.

It was certainly the case with me. Deep inside I knew then that what I was experiencing was much more a spiritual emergency than an emotional one. My vessel was not strong enough to hold all the spiritual information that was flooding me. And I knew it was my spirituality, and only my spirituality, that could save me from the physical and emotional prison that I was in.

You can fight Lyme disease with all the medical expertise available, and I have. You can fortify yourself with the best holistic diet and herbs that money can buy, and I did. I know as sure as I'm writing these words on the page, however, that if you don't have a strong and clear spiritual connection you don't stand a chance against any disease.

Yes, I was saddened by, and furious about, my dad's actions and to be honest, sometimes I'm still angry with him for what he did.

When my heart is clear, however, I know that he saved my life. I also now know that the psych ward was only another step on an intense spiritual-seeking mission.

I had to go through the darkness if I was to shed any light on the disease I didn't even know I had.

I awoke in a strange bed, in a dimly lit room, on a cold December afternoon and I couldn't seem to put the pieces together. I had the feeling in the pit of my stomach that told me to trust no one and get the hell out of wherever I had ended up.

When you are heavily medicated, which I was, it is difficult to tell the difference between a person who is trying to help you and a person who couldn't care less about the amount of psychiatric medications they are pumping into your bloodstream. There are also those people who are interested in the psychotic banter coming out of the heavily medicated person's mouth, and those who nod, stare, and think, *Ohhh boy, this one's gonna take a while to bring back down to earth. Better up her dosage.*

And so it was with my first doctor at Silver Hill Hospital.

Undoubtedly intelligent, Dr. "B" tried to be kind but it was a kindness that I suspect had been eroded by disappointment, life, or maybe his job. He seemed unapproachable, and he was one of the up-the-dose guys. He seemed to have little patience for me and just thought I was completely out of my mind, which I guess I still was—I was still reading people's fortunes with a regular deck of cards.

I was given one of those marble-colored composition books to keep a journal and in it I wrote, "Dr. B is an analytical prick." He was like everybody else in my life who just wouldn't listen to me. I wanted to scream, *I know I'm crazy right now but you wouldn't blame me if I explained it to you!*

My brain had trouble functioning in the best of circumstances, but in the Acute Care Unit of the psychiatric hospital, let's just say it wasn't the perfect setting for clear thinking. I didn't know what to make of my life. So much of it hurt, so much of it was confusing. Yet it also seemed as though I was on a path that had been set long before I was born and it was such a wondrous path, filled with interesting people and exciting places and things. I didn't know why this was all happening to me and therefore couldn't explain it to other people. I was a mouse in a maze.

My mother came to the hospital to visit me. She brought me some warm clothing, sweatshirts, and socks. I'd packed for Jamaica, lots of sarongs and silk cover-ups, and cutoff shorts for the beach—not exactly the appropriate garb for a crazy house in the Connecticut winter. Mom wasn't at all happy with my dad for putting me in a psych ward in the way that he did it, especially without consulting her. She thought he was trying to come up with quick and drastic solutions to fix the problem, a problem that no one could even pinpoint.

In looking back, again, I don't blame my dad. The night I locked myself in the bathroom and asked him to get me pot convinced him that I was addicted to drugs, and he suspected ones much more harmful than marijuana, such as acid or angel dust (PCP), which I have never touched. When you add the ride he took to the Colorado airport with the twelve-step taxi driver, he thought he was doing the right thing. But I don't blame my mother, either. I'd be pissed too if someone abducted my daughter in the middle of the night against her will.

Though I was drugged to my eyelashes and loopy as ever, I somehow knew my mom was on my side. During her visit I was able to articulate that I didn't like my doctor. I told her that the one assigned to me wasn't someone I could open up to or relate to. A suit and a tie and a serious stare only made me want to act crazier than I already was. (I've described how I made him wear the hat with pom-poms on it when he and I had private meetings in my room, remember?) It seemed that he just wanted me to shut up, and I just wanted to get the fuck out of the mental ward.

Unfortunately the crazy in me hadn't left the station yet. Though I was stuck and drugged, I wasn't quite ready to surrender. I begged my mom to spring me. I called lawyers and my friend Danielle and begged them to come get me. My mom told me she couldn't take me home, but she would see if she could get me a different doctor.

It was about this point when I decided to become Chief, the character in *One Flew Over the Cuckoo's Nest*. I kept to myself, said little, and watched. I ate peanut butter out of those little Smucker's packets, which led me to an intense peanut butter addiction, which was helpful, actually, because I'd become so skinny. I barely spoke with any of the patients. The most exciting part of the day was the cigarette break. As if you were in front of a firing squad, they allowed you just one cigarette per break. I would smoke it away from the others by myself.

I robotically complied with the daily routines assigned to the patients in the ACU, mostly group therapies, meals, and arts and crafts or some other type of mindless activity. A nurse named Mary, an Irishwoman, who was actually kind of sweet, told me to take my meds, listen to the doctors, and do as I was told and I'd get out of there quicker. I did it all.

As bleak as things were, I saw a glimmer of light. I'd begun to think about my uncle Billy. Billy always had a place in my thoughts, but I thought of him mostly when I felt lonely or vulnerable. I would talk to him, or pray to him. Soon after I began talking to a male nurse or a nurse's aide, one who came every other Friday. He was large and tall and had long red hair, like my uncle. He was also a musician and would play the acoustic guitar for everyone in the common area.

One day he came into my room and began to talk about Pac-Man. I hadn't mentioned to him that I had a vintage Pac-Mac arcade game in my bedroom at my dad's house, and that I used to stay up until four in the morning high on weed beating my personal best. Yet here he was, sitting on the edge of my bed, randomly comparing Pac-Man to my situation. "You just got to keep eating all the ghosts," he said with a smile that was so familiar it gave me chills. He'd play a guitar outside my room, and I began to believe that I was going to survive. He would joke with me the way my uncle used to. He made me laugh, something refreshingly new.

The hope he brought to me was fleeting, however. I remember looking out of the window of my room when he'd leave me. Through the bars I'd see the desolate winter view and know that people out there were living their lives, going to restaurants and the movies. I wanted to live again.

My spirit was greatly dimmed and saddened. My body was weak, tired. The sensation of bright lights in my eyes was becoming increasingly painful, and I didn't dare tell any of the nurses that loud sounds were starting to hurt my ears. The only fragment of the old me, or the true me, was the wooden painted statue of Ganesh, the magnificent elephant-headed deity, and my favorite lip gloss, which a therapist gave me when she saw that I was desperate for some reminder of my old reality.

In looking back, I was a frightened little girl in Levi's flared jeans, which were a challenge to keep on my hips, and my orange and navy Adidas dunk sneakers, which had my drawings all over them in ball-point pen, and a far-too-large hoodie sweatshirt. That image is certainly not anywhere close to the one depicted on *Rich Girls*.

I've mentioned it was winter. Cold weather was, and still is, a great fear of mine. I wore about six layers of random pieces of clothing. I was adamant about wearing a tight tank top or undershirt, a long-sleeve tee, short-sleeve tee, a sweater, a vest, and a coat. Scarf, hat, gloves were a given. I had perfected the art of socks: Sometimes I'd wear two pair of thin cotton, and other times a heavy wool, depending on the shoes. Cashmere made my feet sweat, and sport socks were not warm enough. It took me a long time to get dressed, configuring all of the layers together like a puzzle so that I would not only be comfortable and warm, but not too hot indoors, and not look like a stuffed sausage. (As a result of Lyme, I still get anxious every time I have to dress or pack for cold weather!)

Although the Chief role remained my default setting, after a week or so in the ACU I did begin to interact with a couple of the other patients. One was a young kid about my age who looked as if he'd done too much ecstasy or acid. We liked to draw together. He was an incredible illustrator—he's probably a tattoo artist now if he isn't dead. In the journal Dr. B had me keep are amazing sketches of mushrooms with human faces my friend drew for me.

I also warmed up to a woman named Giddy, who was a very tall, eccentric character with a huge head of short, dyed red curly hair. She reminded me of Lucille Ball's film version of Auntie Mame, circa 1974. She was glamorous and wore velvet bathrobes. Once a therapist herself, she had entered a deep depression when her son died. I think I was one of the only people to whom she opened up. You know how I got her to do it? I listened. That's all. I was able to do for Giddy what I'd yearned for myself. When you just listen to someone it's amazing what happens.

After about two weeks, the doctor upped my meds to a point where it was difficult for me just to keep my eyes open. I remember thinking I might as well just give in to the power of all the medication. I slept as much as I could. I was dead tired from the meds and the fact that I hadn't slept for the two weeks before I was hospitalized. Now, however, I didn't want to stay awake. There was no reason to. I didn't know what was the matter with me and no one was telling me why I was in the hospital. I cried myself to sleep wishing that I would wake up in my own bed, away from all of this physical and emotional pain.

With each day that passed at Silver Hill I lost more faith. For a while I'd hoped for a hero, perhaps my dad, who would realize his mistake and see things for the way they truly were—I was ill, not crazy. But as time passed my hope dimmed until it was just a dying ember. I began to believe in my heart that no one was riding to my rescue. I don't think I've ever been in such a dark emotional place.

One day about three weeks into my stay at Silver Hill Hospital's Acute Care Unit, the curtains in my dark room were swooshed open with great intention, as if a magician were revealing a trick. It was around seven in the morning and I slowly opened my swollen eyelids to see a woman with wavy chestnut hair, sparkly eyes with purple eye shadow, a long purple silk coat with lots of flowy pink and purple scarves, and more keys on several jingly key rings than a janitor. She was about fifty, my height, and she had a warm smile.

"Good morning Alexandria!" the woman said in a quick, bright way. "How do you feel, sweetie?"

She moved as swiftly as she spoke, and she seemed like a whirlwind of purple and pink jingly dreams, a fairy godmother coming to save me. In fact, for a little while I thought she was a dream. She introduced herself as Dr. Shander. A psychiatrist, she was replacing Dr. B. As it turned out, my mother was the one who had ridden to the rescue and made the hospital change my doctor. She had also given Dr. Shander an earful about my being overmedicated.

In my room that day, Dr. Shander promised that she would get me out of the ACU very soon, which made my heart soar. I didn't even ask her where I would go. I just wanted to leave the unit. She told me that the process of getting me out would speed up if I stopped sleeping so much.

"But I have never felt so tired in my life. All I want to do is sleep," I said.

She promised that she was going to have my meds changed and I would feel a little bit more like my old self. I didn't know what my old self was like at that point. The life I'd left behind seemed so long ago.

Dr. Shander asked me if I knew why I was in the hospital and I told her I had no idea. One of the nurses had said something about PTSD and I thought that maybe I'd experienced some kind of trauma that I didn't remember (which actually wasn't too far off the mark).

"I think I freaked out my dad," I said.

"How did you do that?"

"Channeling Bob Marley and reading too many tarot cards?" (Not to mention the little surprise on the silver tray I handed him.)

The doctor laughed in a way that made me feel safe and called me a "special girl."

She talked to me about my use of alcohol and marijuana and said that there was a lot of marijuana in my system when I came in. She thought maybe some of what I smoked was laced with formaldehyde, which could have flipped my switch and led to psychosis.

"My flip had been switched long before I began smoking pot," I said, and she laughed again. It's only now that I realize how appropriate my statement was.

"Okay, Alexandria, we are going to lower your dosage of medication; you're going to stop sleeping so much, participate in the daily activities, and stop reading tarot cards because it makes you look a little nutty to the nurses. And I'll be back tomorrow!"

As she left my room, Dr. Shander bowed in front of my mini Ganesh statue, which was sitting on top of the desk, and said, "Good morning, Ganesh. Please look after Princess Alexandria today."

And *poof*! The door swung open with her flowing silk coat and tasseled scarves floating behind, and she jingle-jangled away down the hall.

After she left, I fell asleep, and when I awoke again I wasn't sure whether or not I'd dreamed the doctor's visit. My pillow was soaked with sweat, tears, or both and I felt a sense of elation that I hadn't experienced in weeks, maybe months. Although I didn't know it then, Dr. Shander would become my spiritual Sherpa, guiding me through the wilderness and telling me how to face the dragons, how to carry my pack, when to sleep, how to survive in this totally foreign world. She was the one of whom I had my vague dream. She was my phantom healer.

There were only one or two little problems: I was still on just about every psychiatric drug imaginable and I was so weakened by my condition and the medication I could barely get out of bed. And the hospital I was in wasn't treating me for what was really making me sick.

I will tell you this, however. I might have weighed only eighty-seven pounds but I've always been a fighter, and if there was any way for me to fight my way out of the darkness in which I'd been encased, I was about to try my hardest.

sixteen

THE PURPLE GODDESS

"Antibodies to the bacterium that causes Lyme disease have been found in a number of psychiatric patients, suggesting that Lyme disease might trigger psychiatric illness."
—AMERICAN JOURNAL OF PSYCHIATRY

Though I didn't fully know why I was in Silver Hill Hospital, I was so happy to be out of the ACU that it really didn't matter. Earlier I packed my things and was driven by a white van the fifty yards that separated the buildings. We pulled up to Barrett House which looked like a traditional early American home with charming windows and pretty landscaping. As I approached the home-style door, I was looking forward to being in a place that didn't have bars on the windows and hospital corridors. I was taken to a room with two beds, so I knew I had a roommate. Not the most ideal situation, but anything was better than sleeping where I had been.

After I put my stuff in the room, a counselor led me to a living room, where I sat on a caramel-colored wooden chair with an oversize back. Surrounding me were women of all different ages who sat on a couch, armchairs, a rocking chair, or folding chairs; one person was sprawled out on the floor. My joints were aching, and I couldn't sit comfortably in any chair; therefore I was fidgety. Thank goodness the chair on which I sat at least had a cushion. I didn't care that it was mauve, stained, and lumpy; I just didn't want it to squeak while readjusting.

A woman walked into the room who looked like she had been working there for quite a while. She had on a peach sweater, pleated khakis, and gold-rimmed glasses. "Okay, ladies, we are going to fill out a PTSD packet today. Does anybody know what PTSD is?" The woman was chipper, yet firm and meant business. She reminded me of one of my math teachers in sixth grade at the Convent of the Sacred Heart.

A woman in her late forties with bushy blond-grayish hair, skinny legs, and a large gut raised her hand. She was wearing baggy teal leggings and a pale yellow turtleneck. Her face was red and bloated and she looked as if she hadn't slept for days. I didn't know where any of these women came from, why we were all here, and what we were doing. "I'm a nurse," the lady said, "so I am very familiar with post-traumatic stress disorder."

Naturally, I thought the group therapy session I'd joined was about PTSD. Both Dr. Shander and the nurses in the ACU had mentioned that I might be suffering from post-traumatic stress. As I sat there, however, I realized that PTSD was not the main focus of the discussion. We had to fill out a pamphlet that asked questions like "When was your first drink or drug?" or "Do you black out when you drink?"

Why do they want to know about drinking? I wondered.

In looking back, I know it seems crazy (pun intended) that it took me so long to realize I was in an alcohol and drug rehab. You have to remember, though, they were still pumping me with all sorts of meds, even antipsychotics. You could have asked me who was the president of the United States and I might have gotten it wrong. But also, my alcohol and drug use wasn't at the top of the list of things I thought I had a problem with.

As a seventeen- and eighteen-year-old, I partied with the best of my peer group, even drank some college kids under the table. At times, did I drink too much? You betcha. Smoke too much pot? Yup, yup. But I never felt as though I was addicted to alcohol or pot. I was attempting to ease the pain I was in. I used pot and alcohol more as a misguided attempt to feel normal. That's all I really wanted—to feel normal and not hurt.

On the questionnaire, I wrote that I *needed* to smoke pot. I had insomnia, my joints and muscles were in constant agony, I frequently felt nauseated. Pot soothed my stomach, gave me an appetite, and helped with my headaches, I wrote.

I looked around the room, and some women were crying while writing their answers. I finally put the pieces together: This house was for women who abused alcohol and drugs, and my doctor thought I was one of them. I was freaked out and confused. I was paranoid that I had pulled the wool over my own eyes and was perhaps in deep denial that I had a real alcohol or drug addiction problem. It messed with my head.

I knew I was in no condition to tell them that I didn't think I belonged. So I gave in to the circumstance. I decided I'd just ride out whatever this was and hope for the chance to talk to someone who could get a little better sense of what was going on with me.

After that first group session, I found myself in the sunny backyard of the hospital's Barrett House. Still layered in multiple items of ill-fitting clothing, I felt comforted knowing that I could go outside and sit on the gray wooden bench to stare at the little creek while sucking down as many cigarettes as I could. Just having fresh air to breathe, albeit laced with Marlboro Light smoke, while letting the warm sun rest on my face felt a little closer to freedom.

The creek reminded me of one near Nonnie's house. My cousin Mike Fredo had placed troll dolls in the roots and hollows of the trees that grew near the brook. It was like a little troll town. I wanted to live in a tree like the trolls, and when I was little, every time I came upon a tree hollow enough to hold me I'd climb in and feel warm and safe. Outside the Barrett House that first day, my heart and soul still felt numb, probably number than in the ACU, but being around nature brought back happy childhood memories of running around in the forest behind my houses in Greenwich. The peace and stillness made me feel settled.

The fact was, though, I wanted to say in the worst way, "Get me off whatever you have stifling my personality, and I'll be your best friend forever." Instead, I just kept taking the goddamn meds in fear that I would be locked back up in the ACU if I didn't.

In the backyard of Barrett House I felt the same way about telling anyone that I didn't think I was an alcoholic or drug addict. I was afraid if I did they would send me back to the ACU.

Later that day, I met with the senior social worker, a woman in her sixties who looked friendly. As I walked into her tiny office filled with little dried bouquets of roses and porcelain tea cups, tears began to swell as I realized that she had a life on the outside, and there was life beyond the lock and key of this institution. Maybe this woman would have a heart. Maybe she would understand that I really didn't need to be here.

My plea and cry to go home did not work. She saw through me like a CT scan! She grinned and nodded and listened. She didn't say much. She actually pretended to consider my request, which did give me a glimmer of hope. I was so desperate to go home. I was still walking around with what felt like Vaseline smeared in my eyes. My brain was pure butter, and ice encased my heart and soul. I couldn't feel feelings or express any joy or even sadness anymore, except at night in bed when I would cry. I could barely process the information they were giving me, and I wasn't good at making friends because I was still acting like Chief. I only let my guard down with Giddy, who seemed to have compassion for me and what I was going through.

I was grateful to be in a proper bedroom, though, even one with a roommate. She seemed like a sweet girl around my age. Her parents had taken her out of college to come here, and I think she was just as confused as I was. She was petite like me, too, with red hair and freckles. She knew how to knit, which I thought was cool, and she made really pretty scarves with gold thread throughout the weave. I was confused as to why she was in this hospital, because she seemed so normal. There was no way she had a drug or alcohol problem.

But I was terrified she'd seen *Rich Girls* and was going to tell the rest of the women in the house. Though the meds had reduced my obsession with the show, the thought of it would invade my mind every now and then with the force of a terrible army. When those invasions happened, I would literally wince from the pain and embarrassment.

When I left the senior social worker's office I knew I was trapped, and that first night underneath three blankets I buried my head in the scratchy pillow and wept. I felt as if I were in an alternate universe, trapped in a net of nothingness.

The next day, it was a challenge for me to wake up at 7 a.m. I felt so drained and my hands were so swollen that I couldn't bend them, which I didn't know then is very common with people suffering from Lyme (ask a Lyme sufferer about how long it takes to button a shirt!). The size of my hands was surprising and a little scary.

At seven thirty we gathered in the living area and went around the room and read from a meditation book. I didn't understand a word that was being read, and I didn't care. I wanted to go back to bed. When it came my turn to read, I thought my heart was going to jump out of my throat. I knew I couldn't put a sentence together, let alone read out loud in front of a room of women. I used to be able to put my acting hat on and just read with ease and a bit of charisma. But that instinct had vanished and I tripped over the words as though I had a mouth filled with crackers. I was humiliated, and after the fourth line of the paragraph decided to pass.

As the days crawled by, I began to fully comprehend that not only was I in a drug and alcohol rehabilitation center, but I was in one that was well known in the field of recovery. Famous patients the center had treated included Judy Garland (and her daughter Liza Minnelli), Truman Capote, Joan Kennedy, and Gregg Allman. I liked the fact that Gregg Allman and Truman Capote had been there—that was something I could wear with pride.

My class at the Silver Hill academy had its own characters.

There was a Puerto Rican woman I'll call "Leddy" who was a Lexapro poster child. She just loved the fact that the antidepressant was working for her. Her history was one of locking herself in her apartment, putting black plastic garbage bags over her windows, and smoking pot for weeks at a time. There was a girl named Steph who had lived in the Barrett House for more than a year. You couldn't tell Steph was a girl unless she took off her hat and let down her hair. She was tough, guarded, and knew the ropes.

There was the nurse and now patient named Dotty, who was bloated and had fried, curly hair. There was a mother of three young children who was a crack and meth head, and there was a woman who looked like a real estate agent from Fort Lauderdale, with bleached-blond hair, hot pink long fingernails, and frosted lipstick; she wore a lot of exercise clothes. She kind of figured out who I was and became very friendly. Months later, someone would tell me that she got drunk and drowned in her Jacuzzi.

There were two or three other younger women with whom I became friendly over time. Christie was a smart and sarcastic New Jersey chick who really wanted what the rehab offered her. Kerry had dark Irish looks, a wicked sense of humor, and a bad case of OCD—her hands were always red and cracked from being washed. And there was Joanie. About my age, Joanie was a beautiful, free-spirited, hippy, bisexual ex–heroin addict.

In time I began to fall into the routine of the center and found that I really liked the structure. For so much of my life, certainly for the previous year or so, structure was something that had been sorely missing. In a way, the rehab routine was like going to the college I'd never been to.

Every morning I met with the others in the living room to see the schedule for the day. Then it was on to the cafeteria to eat breakfast. After breakfast, some patients would go to an AA meeting in a church in New Canaan. People from the meeting would come pick them up and drop them off. I went to a few in my first days in rehab and found that I didn't relate with anyone. The AA meetings outside the rehab were filled with older women. The way they talked about *having* to drink alcohol kind of creeped me out. So instead of the meeting, I had free time after breakfast and I'd go out to the backyard and smoke and try to figure out how to strategically layer my clothing for the day.

The rest of the day was filled with group therapy, lunch, free time, group therapy, an AA meeting in the rehab, dinnertime in the cafeteria, free time, and finally bed. The groups were titled Self-Esteem and Setting Daily Goals. Though I liked to smoke my American Spirits (I had switched from Marlboro Lights), I wasn't fond of the free time so I became very regimented. It was as if I was holding on to the daily structure for fear of spinning off into space if I didn't.

Like a purple tornado, Dr. Shander came in twice a week to visit me. Shander is quick and smart and a doer, and initially at rehab I was put off by her energy. I thought I needed a bit more of the calming, nurturing type. I was a damaged and delicate butterfly and would recoil from anyone who was even the slightest bit abrupt.

To Shander I complained that having a roommate made me feel uncomfortable. I was still worried about the fallout from the TV show and that the gossip columns would find out I was in a drug-and-alcohol rehab facility. My roommate had mentioned that she'd seen the show and I got a little freaked out. I just couldn't handle the raw feelings I still had from *Rich Girls*.

But the main reason I wanted to be on my own was that I was embarrassed—I was crying myself to sleep every night. I felt trapped and lonely and depressed. I wasn't able to socialize properly. I'd spent so much time putting on a brave face and not showing people how I was feeling, there wasn't a lot of room for my true emotions. I didn't know how to show people how I felt.

"Ally, walk toward things that make you happy and feel good," Shander would say, "and walk away from things that make you feel bad or are negative. You have all the answers, choose wisely."

Maybe my lowest emotional point at Silver Hill was the day my boyfriend Charlie came to visit. He had been with me throughout the breakdown. Our relationship was sweet and innocent, but it had since faded.

I told Charlie I couldn't see him anymore because I had nothing to give. What I really meant was, *I have absolutely no physical, emotional, or mental capacity right now, and I do not know how to be a girlfriend, or even a human. Don't let me traumatize you any further, and don't try to touch me or kiss me because I can't feel it.* I couldn't stand stringing him along, especially without being able to feel any emotions. (What I didn't know then was that sexual attraction in Lyme patients runs to both ends of the spectrum: Either you lack sexual drive, or you can't get enough sex. I'd experience both. In Silver Hill, I was at the lowest end of the spectrum.)

Charlie was a really good guy. I hadn't let the relationship fall into any sort of intimacy when we were together; we were more like best friends who made out. I felt that he deserved more. It was sad, and one of us cried. When he drove off, I wondered if I had done the right thing.

I truly wondered if I would ever be well enough to love anyone.

Again, like Chief from *One Flew Over the Cuckoo's Nest,* with the little canvas jacket he wore that was a bit too small for him (mine was corduroy with a bit of shearling at the collar), I stared into space, into the abyss of fear and nothingness, wondering when my brain would return from wherever it was being kept.

It was around this time that I told Dr. Shander that I thought I needed to see a different doctor. She was bombarding me with questions, like where I would live when I left, which were unmanageable for me at the time. She saw me as a much stronger and more capable person than I felt, so I told her that maybe I needed to switch doctors. I'd begun to form a dependence on the rehab and I was frightened of change.

Dr. Shander asked me why I wanted to switch doctors. That was the scariest scenario: having to be honest and up front with someone as to why I didn't want to see them anymore. I was so unable to sugarcoat anything or process more than what I wanted to have for lunch, so I just told her the truth: "I don't think I can handle all your opinions; it feels overwhelming to me. It's too much at once. I need to find my own opinions."

She smiled and giggled a bit, something I did not expect.

"Ally, of course you should learn to honor your own opinions. In fact, this is a wonderful opportunity for you to really step up to your own inner strength. Anything that interferes with your magnificence is going to make you small. So if you want to give us another chance, let's work on you getting rid of your obstacles and living your own inner power."

I was hesitant, but after all she was the one who had saved me from the ACU. So I agreed to continue. I am so grateful I did give her another chance, because it turned out to be one of the most impactful relationships of my life.

seventeen

NIGHTS IN WHITE SATIN

*"You cannot travel the path until you
have become the path itself."*
—BUDDHA

One morning I walked into the dimly lit living area, which had one couch, a rocking chair, two armchairs with Cornwall blue velvet fabric that had slightly faded in the back from the afternoon sun, and another large armchair with torn cream linen and a doily. *Why do people use doilies?* I wondered. *Why would someone put mauve floral print fabric on a couch?* It was what hung above the couch, however, that caught my attention.

I imagine that the sign had been hanging there since Judy Garland had sat on the mauve floral print, but it was as if it had magically appeared that morning. I just hadn't noticed it at all. The words in the picture frame read: "God, grant me the serenity to accept the things I cannot change, the courage to change the things I can, and the wisdom to know the difference."

It's not as though I had some type of white-light spiritual experience that morning. As a matter of fact, the "God" part of the prayer bothered me. It brought back memories of the Convent of Sacred

Heart and being told what I had to believe in. I had not believed in Catholicism's idea of God in a long time. I'd jumped that ship for good when I was thirteen and refused to be confirmed in the Catholic Church. Besides, I was so furious at humans creating death, destruction, and war over religion and God. It was too hypocritical.

But the idea of acceptance, the courage to change, and the sense to figure things out began to find a foothold in the mushy walls of my brain. As the days went by, the Serenity Prayer became a mantra that would help quiet my thoughts and give me strength. I still wasn't sold on the God thing, at least not the one with the flowing robe and long, white beard, but someone told me that it could be a god of my understanding, like a tree or Ganesh, and that made it a little easier for me to believe.

The other thing I wasn't sold on was that I was an alcoholic or drug addict. It was Steph who told me that I'd better act like I was sold on it or else they wouldn't let me out. She knew from experience, she said. I suppose she was once in my shoes, and desperately wanted to leave, and realized she might as well accept the fact that she was there. She realized later that the rehab was a safe and reliable place for her and she grew more comfortable there. Little did I know, the same thing would happen to me.

My days were filled with monotonous tasks that I began to enjoy doing, like making my bed and going to the gym and to the dining hall at the same times every day. I enjoyed the monotony, I think, because I could concentrate on a task without having to make many decisions. If I went to the gym, I would alternately stare at the treadmill, the elliptical machine, and the stationary bike. It would take me fifteen minutes just to decide on which machine to work out. Making decisions took up most of my workout time.

And back in my room, I had only two pairs of jeans, a couple of sweaters, and about four shirts, but you'd think I had a wardrobe to fill a walk-in closet. *Should I put on the long-sleeve shirt or the short-sleeve shirt? Do I need a sweater? Or is the shearling corduroy jacket enough? Maybe just a puffy vest over a sweater?* I'd stand in my room looking at my clothes as if they were an unsolvable riddle.

Whatever I wore needed to have pockets somewhere to hold my American Spirits and the little red-coral statue of Buddha sitting by his tree stump that I carried with me everywhere I went. I'd found the Buddha at a Tibetan antique shop on Bleecker Street in New York City one day while I was waiting to meet a friend for coffee.

The little Buddha made the trip to Silver Hill and now when I touched it I could almost feel the old me that had been left behind. I kept the statuette with me everywhere I went and would reach for it when I needed to feel grounded or comforted.

Though clothing and workout choices still stymied me, I did appreciate tasks that required no thought at all. That was a huge benefit of being in rehab.

One day I couldn't find the little Buddha. I enlisted the entire population of Barrett House, patients and staff, to look for it. I don't remember where Leddy found it, but when she did, I laughed with relief and hugged her, which took everyone by surprise. Except for the soft weeping into my pillow, the only emotion I'd shown up until then was the "Mmmmm . . ." I purred when I was eating my peanut butter packets.

I had never been fond of peanut butter before, but now it was the one thing I looked forward to in the evening. I must have downed a half a jar of Skippy crunchy peanut butter every single night. I became a bit concerned about the peanut butter intake when I had a hard time fitting into my jeans, and I could now handle only four layers of clothing instead of six. I asked to see a nutritionist for fear that I had contracted some sort of eating disorder.

The nutritionist looked as if she could use some daily doses of peanut butter herself, and maybe a few hamburgers. She told me that for someone my height, I should be consuming about twelve hundred calories per day. I just gave up on the whole nutritionist thing—I couldn't add up the calories anyhow—and decided I was not going to become neurotic about my unusual eating habits. I felt liberated. Vive la peanut butter!

To my surprise, each day my mood improved a little.

Dr. Shander had kept her promise and kept lowering the medication until I was finally weaned off everything I had been taking. Without the lead feet and the cobwebbed thoughts that came with the meds, I actually began to feel at home at Barrett House, and I began to grow fond of the doilies and faded velvet fabric. The smell of crappy burnt coffee brewing in the kitchen actually made me feel cozy and safe.

The big moment came when I moved into a private room, which was part of a deal Dr. Shander and I made when she convinced me I needed to stay in the house for a while longer. Maybe it was a bit self-centered of me, or maybe I was still paranoid about the TV show, but as nice as my roommate was I had trouble falling asleep because I felt as if she might be watching my every move. It didn't help that I had absolutely no boundaries and I was always lending her sweaters and products. She did the bathroom cleaning, though, and I was happy to lend a few sweaters instead of swabbing the toilet.

A funny thing happened when I moved into the private room. I actually became obsessed with cleaning! I spent hours scrubbing that bathroom from top to bottom. Up until then, I don't think I'd ever cleaned a bathroom in my life. You know something? That's not cool. Everybody should know the satisfaction of doing your own cleaning and keeping your own house.

I just went all in with had a room full of suds and water and scrubbed. I did this in my underwear so I wouldn't get my clothes all wet. I had fun, and I now appreciate a clean bathroom. I also learned how to do laundry properly. My mother had taught me how to iron and how to wash the dishes but had never really explained separating laundry. I used to throw all of it in at once, sprinkle in some powdered detergent (whatever was in the blue box above the antique washer), and press start. When my clothes came out bleached, faded, and shrunken, a woman in Barrett House noticed that I had transformed half of my wardrobe into tie-dye baby clothes. Right then and there, she taught me the basics of sorting through my clothes and how to do laundry properly.

Learning how to clean and to manage my own laundry helped me feel like I was growing up, and becoming a normal human being among other normal human beings (whatever normal means). It was a step toward maturity, being grounded, and independence.

The weeks became months at Barrett House, and I to started feel comfort and confidence in the routine. I believe this came from my Swiss-German background on my father's side of the family.

Being off all the meds had one big downside, though. I began to feel the pain in my joints again, especially in my knees, which began to swell and throb. One day, I found a branch in the woods behind Barrett House and used it as a walking stick. Holding it made me feel both steady on my feet and spiritually grounded. In one way, the stick represented a full circle for me: from the midst of my breakdown in the tree near the Orlando airport to walking the grounds of Silver Hill with a branch that made me feel almost whole again.

I was walking with the stick one day when a new girl approached me. She was drop-dead gorgeous, a model no doubt. Yikes! With the way I looked and in this dreadful place I was so frightened of meeting people in fashion. I didn't want to see anyone from "my world." My vanity dissipated when the new girl came up to me more interested in my new walking stick than in my overly washed flared Levi's.

"That's a cool stick. Where did you find it?" she asked ever so confidently.

"I just found it out by the creek. I think it's pretty cool. It reminds me of an old man. It has the personality of an old man who lives in a cabin in the woods, you know?"

"I know exactly what you mean! You're so right, it totally does." From them on, this woman and I began one of my favorite friendships. Her name is Courtney, or Coco for short.

We walked to the group meeting that evening with my walking stick in hand and began singing the Moody Blues song "Nights in White Satin." It was totally random, but somehow I knew in that moment that I had turned the corner on my spiritual path. I was finally coming back into my body. My soul was returning.

By the end of February, the middle-aged social worker with all the dried roses gave me passes to go home a couple of times. I stayed at my mother's house, because it was the place where I felt most comfortable. I freaked out the first time I was there, seeing all of the Christmas gifts I didn't open, the writing on the walls of my art studio during my psychotic break, and all of the memories came flooding back. I realized how out there I was before I came into the rehab, how unmanageable my life had become. I was a different person staring into the bathroom mirror near where I used to roll my nightly joints. It brought up triggering thoughts and it was emotional for me. On one of these visits I was reunited with my car, which I brought back to the rehab. And in February, on my nineteenth birthday, my dad came to pick me up and took me out to a steak dinner in Stamford. My parents tried to make the occasion as happy as they could. They brought balloons and my mom brought me a goldfish (my mom sometimes had a strange idea of what would make me happy; one Easter she dyed my Westie dog, Sally, pink).

At my birthday dinner, I sat across from Dad as if I were in a confessional. At meetings and group, we'd begun to talk about the twelve steps—I was following what everyone else was doing. I knew that the steps were partly about taking accountability for what you'd done. "I'm really sorry if I said or did anything to hurt you," I said to him sincerely. "I smoked pot, drank, and I have done cocaine a couple of times." He was sweet and let me off the hook easily. I returned to the rehab that night filled with happiness and hope. I didn't have to say anything to my mother, because she was just so loving and understanding when she came to visit. She honestly didn't think I needed to be there or going to twelve-step meetings. Looking back, I think the program provided me an opportunity to heal, meet great people, mature, and be really honest with myself. Maybe I didn't have the classic case of "alcoholism," but somehow I knew that being sober was going to offer me a solid strength that I would need when going through a totally different type of healing.

It was in the spring, the time for rebirth and new beginnings, when Dr. Shander came into my room, calmly this time, and sat on the bed across from me. "Ally, sweetie, you have been here for three and a half months. You are doing so well, it's amazing how much you have improved since you got here. It's time for you to go and live in the real world."

I was shocked. I didn't know how to react. I had been home three or four times on weekend passes, but I always enjoyed coming back to Barrett House. The scratchy sheets and lumpy pillows didn't bother me anymore, and it became an easy ritual to wake up at six thirty and have bland boiled eggs and oatmeal.

"But Dr. Shander, I don't know if I'm really ready. What if I break down? Where should I live? What will I do with my days?"

"I know you're ready mostly because you do not want to leave, and that's a sign that someone needs to start a new life. Can you get a job somewhere?"

I'd thought about this already, and my mother had offered me a little job at her company, the children's clothing store on Greenwich Avenue called Best & Company. It was by far the chicest store in town. She offered to let me work upstairs in the design room and assist the designers. I told Dr. Shander.

"Well, that sounds great!" she responded. "You will come to my office twice a week, and everything will be fine. I believe in you. You have such a great life to live ahead of you, let's get it going already!"

I was paralyzed with fear. I fought to stay. But Dr. Shander insisted I only had three days left.

"But where will I live?"

Mom and Dad still lived directly across the street from one another: Mom in Denbigh Farm, and Dad behind the fence that looked the same as the Denbigh Farm fence in a house called Appleyard. Dr. Shander and I discussed which place would provide me with the healthiest environment. Both had historical significance, of course, and much of it bad. I'd experienced bleak moments of my breakdown in both. My mom's house, however, felt like more of a threat to my newly sober (marijuana-free) way of life because of all the time I felt alone in it. I'd spent so many days in my room painting and smoking pot, with my mom invisible behind her closed office door. We worried that I would fall back to the same old habit there. We decided that Dad's was the best of two imperfect choices.

As I packed up my room, I realized that I had actually been at the hospital for four months altogether. When all my little knick-knacks had been cleaned off the dresser, and the lovely sheer green fabric my mother had brought for me to put over my bed to add color got folded up, it looked like a hospital again, sad and depressing. I still hated to leave. I put all of my belongings in my car.

When I looked at myself in the rearview mirror, a different person looked back at me. Long gone were the thread-weaved dreads; instead my hair was washed, shiny, and freshly cut. The skin on my face was clear with the natural glow of a nineteen-year-old. I had gained a few pounds thanks to Skippy peanut butter and it suited me. I was no longer sluffing around in sweatpants or ill-fitting Levi's but was wearing dark denim jeans. The thought of *Rich Girls* now was almost completely gone from my mind.

I was frightened about the future. I was also worried about how I felt physically and mentally. Some days everything felt fine and then, wham, my knees would be killing me and my brains would be scrambled. I was still waking up in drenched sheets on the nights when I could actually fall asleep. There were days toward the end of my time at Barrett House when the pain was worse than ever. I kept my symptoms from Dr. Shander because I was already so overwhelmed just figuring out how to navigate rehab. The only symptoms I ever explained to her were the intense fatigue I was experiencing.

The day I left rehab, I started my car and drove straight to Dr. Shander's office for our first appointment outside of the hospital. I had no way of knowing, of course, that I was leaving Silver Hill with the same disease I had when I was put into the ACU.

part three

eighteen

THE BATTLE BEGINS

"Lyme disease can mimic many psychiatric and cognitive disorders, and increase the severity of prior underlying symptoms."
—RICHARD HOROWITZ, M.D.

Don't you love it when life is going by so easily and happily, and it's springtime, the trees have blossomed, the sun is shining, your car is running smoothly, the sound of the birds makes your heart skip beats, you get to places on time, you smile at the barista genuinely and gladly, and then BAM, you get hit on top of the head by a giant green monster that has been following you, waiting for the perfect opportunity to hit you, maybe while you're about to sip on your piping hot soy latte?

In my case, I needed the hit. I needed to face the looming, dark figure and say, "Listen, buddy, I know you have been there all along. I could feel your dirty whiskers scratching my face, I can smell your stinky breath, I can sense your impending doom, but I am glad to finally meet you and I am ready to fight!"

At this point in my life, newly released from rehab, I was ill-equipped for the fight. First of all, I didn't know with whom I was fighting; my stay at Silver Hill hadn't addressed my primary disease at all. And second, I was battling this green monster alone. I looked around and asked myself: *Where's my moat, my dragon, my prince, my bows and arrows, my horse, and my squire to guide me through this thorny forest?*

All I had was Dr. Shander, and thank you, Ganesh, for that.

I've described how, while I was still in Silver Hill, Dr. Shander and I decided that my best course of action was to live with my dad at Appleyard and go to work for my mom at Best & Company, her store in Greenwich. So each day I pulled myself out of bed, showered, and dressed. I wore frilly blouses and nice tight jeans and pointy-toed stilettos. I wanted to look my best, and I wanted to get back to work.

At the end of Greenwich Avenue, in a large building with massive cement pillars in front, Best & Company was an awesome store. It was huge and packed with children's clothing, bassinettes, and hobbyhorses. There were antique rugs on the floor and cabinets made of mahogany and brass. My mom hired one of our former housekeepers, an older English woman, to open the door for customers. The customers loved her accent. "Gooooood aaaaftarnooon," she'd say, "welcome to Best and Company."

The design studio and offices were on the second level. I was an assistant to an assistant designer, or at the level of an intern, and I was grateful for it. The designers would give me tasks like pulling out all the raspberry fabric swatches from the bins. I worked hard, and Mom paid me a small salary in a check that the accountant would bring to my desk. The accountant even walked me to the Bank of America, where I opened my first real checking account.

Mom also sent me on a sample shopping trip or two and I visited many children's clothing stores. I really had fun.

I kept my life simple, which helped with my transition back into the real world. I went to some twelve-step meetings and liked the camaraderie and community they offered, though I still didn't feel as though I fit in. There were few people my age at the meetings and I'd find myself spending my nights with older women at diners or playing Balderdash and Pictionary in someone's living room, which isn't exactly a twenty-year-old's idea of excitement.

I also saw Dr. Shander twice a week. It was during one of these early visits with Shander that I received the most important diagnosis of my life.

Filled with crystals and antique wooden statues of ancient goddesses and flowers, usually lilies, Dr. Shander's office had once been someone's pottery studio. It had skylights and a sliding glass door so you could see the trees that surrounded her house with interwoven branches that felt to me like a protective casing. I felt safe in that room. I knew this woman was on my side, that she respected me in a way that no other adult had. Dr. Shander listened to what I said to her about my life, how I was feeling, or about my family, with great concern and compassion. I suppose most therapists listen to their patients in the same manner, but I felt a connection with her like I had with no one else. It was as though I had finally met someone who could see inside of me and maybe, just maybe, the person who could tell me what was wrong in there.

I'd just come from work that day, so I had on makeup and a nice outfit, a flirty skirt and heels. I was telling Dr. Shander how much I loved working for my mom, and how much fun it was to work with children's clothing and colors and fabrics again.

"It's amazing how three weeks ago you couldn't imagine being out of Silver Hill," she said. "You were like a frightened little chick needing to leave the nest, and now you are dressing up every day and going into work! It's awesome, and I am so proud of you."

After being quite positive and complimentary she gave me one of her *Now tell me what's really going on* looks. She was always able to cut through the bullshit that I made myself believe.

It wasn't that I was lying about loving the job and being back in the real world; I was truly grateful and happy about that. What I wasn't telling her, though, was that I felt shitty just about all the time.

My whole body hurt, and even scarier, my brain function was still failing.

"Why didn't you tell me you were feeling so bad?" she asked.

Tears began to well up as the words started billowing out. I told her that I was afraid to say anything because I thought she wouldn't believe me. I thought she'd feel as everyone else did, that I was exaggerating. There were times I wouldn't even go out of the house, I said, because I was afraid I'd run into someone I knew and forget their name. I had already seen so many doctors, and they had given me all sorts of scary diagnoses, brushed me off, or given me medication that never worked. I explained that when I was seven years old, I was diagnosed with "growing pains," and then at eleven with adolescent rheumatoid arthritis, and then they said it might be multiple sclerosis. When I was sixteen the diagnosis was fibromyalgia. I was placed in Silver Hill partly because my dad thought I was a drug addict.

"I hate sounding like a whiner, or someone who can't handle stuff," I said. I sat there with mascara-colored tears running down my face. My faucet was now open and the truth was pouring out.

"I wake up in a pool of sweat every morning," I said between sobs. "I get up in the middle of the night and usually can't get back to sleep. Sometimes my legs hurt so much it feels like someone is sticking knives into my thighs. At work I feel so dumb. My words come out backward, and I can't remember anything. It's so embarrassing. I still can't make a stupid fucking decision on anything! It takes me so long that I forget what I was even supposed to be deciding on in the first place.

"My vision keeps going in and out. I almost crashed getting off of I-95 because I couldn't read the signs. I'm nauseous and have these weird headaches that come every Wednesday at around three o'clock. Every Wednesday! How fucking random is that? I don't have an appetite, and I just know in my gut that something is seriously wrong with me. And this has been going on for years and years and no one has really been able to understand or do anything!"

As I finished pouring out my heart, I took a long, deep breath of relief.

Dr. Shander paused and straightened her purple silk blouse. "Ally, have you been tested for Lyme disease?" she asked.

"Like three or four times," I said. I told her about the specialist in Boston who said the levels weren't quite high enough for him to be able to fully diagnose the disease. They were a half a point short of Lyme disease on the CDC's scale. The way I understand it, the CDC interprets whether or not you have Lyme from the number of bands on the scale of the Western Blot Test. The Western Blot measures antibodies that are problematic in the blood. You are supposed to have five bands for Lyme, and I had four and a half. He said my results were too borderline and the test was inconclusive.

"He told me it was fibromyalgia," I said.

"Do you remember being bit by a tick?" she asked.

"Yes, on the stomach, when I was seven," I said. "Right next to my birthmark." I told Shander how my mother followed the instructions carefully, how she took the tick off with a tweezers and took it to be tested. "They said it wasn't infected."

"You need to listen to me very carefully, Ally," Dr. Shander said. "I think you have Lyme disease, and I think you need to start treating it immediately."

"But tests—the doctors—how could they all be wrong?"

She told me that she'd seen patients who have been suffering terribly with undiagnosed Lyme for years, ones who had been to five, six different doctors who didn't recognize what they had. "These patients come to me with depression, anxiety," she said. "They complain of joint pain, nausea, and horrible headaches. They tell me they have trouble making the simplest decisions. My God. We live in Connecticut, in the middle of Lyme country, and during an epidemic! Lyme should have been the first thing the doctors thought of!"

Shander went on to tell me about the difficulties of diagnosing Lyme, about all the false positives and false negatives, and about the inherent bias against Lyme diagnoses within the medical community. It was confusing, but there was also a flicker of hope in what she said.

I wanted to believe that there was a name to what was wrong with me, and Shander was the first doctor to say there just might be.

"What about Silver Hill, and the way I acted before I was put there?" I asked.

"I've seen Lyme symptoms look psychotic," she said, "and why not? It's an invasion of the brain."

Dr. Shander told me to go to a Dr. Steven Phillips in Danbury, Connecticut. "He will be able to read through your blood work and see what's really going on. It sounds as though you have been suffering for quite some time."

At that moment I didn't realize the enormity of what a Lyme diagnosis would mean to my life; I just remember the comfort and validation her words offered me.

"You have all the symptoms," she said. "I would be shocked if you didn't have it."

Dr. Shander was doctor No. 1. I would see eleven more in my battle against Lyme.

nineteen

IN THE BLOOD

The very next day, I gathered the courage to call Dr. Phillips (doctor No. 2). I'd awakened that morning in sheets that were wringing wet and with swollen fingers. On the phone, Phillips seemed straightforward, earnest, and very smart. I didn't tell him much, just that Dr. Shander had recommended him. We made an appointment for the following week. Shander put in a special call for me to get in right away. Over those next seven days I kept track of how I felt every day and wrote it down. I didn't exaggerate. I just wanted my symptoms on paper so I could show them to the doctor in black-and-white.

As it happened, the Lyme symptoms flared as if the disease knew I was getting ready to fight it.

When the day of the appointment came, I drove to Dr. Phillips's office—well, I actually kind of raced to Dr. Phillip's office. Having learned how to drive from my dad, who is a maniac behind the wheel, and how not to drive from my mom, who likes to drive on the left side of the road "because it feels more British," I'm a defensive but aggressive driver. This day I really had the pedal to the metal. I didn't know what to expect, but I was excited at the prospect of finally finding out what was wrong with me. I sang Neil Young songs all the way, at the top of my lungs.

I'd always relied on my parents to arrange for doctors and to take me to the appointments. I didn't have any say in choosing them, except to say I didn't like going to them, but this time I'd taken charge of my own destiny. My experience in the rehab and my relationship with Dr. Shander had given me this. It felt really good. I did let my parents know about the appointment and they respected the fact that I was taking the reins. I told them I needed to do this for myself. It is always easier to speak to a doctor alone behind closed doors anyhow.

In the middle of belting out "Harvest Moon," I realized that I had passed the office and totally lost track of the directions. I retraced my steps and made about three U-turns before spotting the teeny, tiny structure off the main road. I parked and slowly climbed out. Some of the enthusiasm I'd built on the drive over disappeared when I saw the building. It looked like a prefab house that had been plopped onto a dirt lot on the side of Route 1.

Inside, I sat on a wooden chair in a foyer while my mind wandered and started to conger dark scenarios. *Where am I? A stranger's house where he takes people's blood and analyzes it? Maybe he drinks it and bathes his children in it.*

The doctor hurried down the stairs in old L.L. Bean cargo shorts, a pair I'm sure my father hadn't invented, and an oatmeal and olive plaid short-sleeved camping shirt. He wore hiking boots with those itchy thick wool nubby socks sticking out the top. He was clean-cut, younger than I expected, probably in his early forties, and he had a vibrancy about him that made me wonder if he in fact had been drinking the blood upstairs.

Probably out of a stainless steel thermos.

I followed him down the hallway to an office that was top-to-bottom pine, like some secret log cabin laboratory. *Would this guy really know what to do if he found anything wrong with me?* I wondered. I kept reminding myself that Dr. Shander recommended him. Fake flowers, knotty pine, and L.L. Bean aside, he had to be good.

His office was in a rather small room. It had one simple desk, again wood, like the desk that a third-grade teacher would have in her classroom. I sat in one of the two generic chairs in front of his desk. The desk was covered in files and papers and folders. *This is good,* I thought. *He must be some type of busy genius.* I'd seen so many doctors already in my short life that I'd honed a sharp instinct about them. It was like *Name That Tune.* I could tell in a couple of notes if my heart felt safe, and warm.

Dr. Phillips wasn't big on chitchat. After an exchange of a few pleasantries about Shander and my ride over, he got right to the point. "Tell me why you're here."

My main complaint, I told him, the one that had lasted the longest and stayed the most consistently, was joint pain, the worst of it coming in my hips and knees.

He then asked me something that no one had ever asked me before: "Does it ever jump around? Is it sometimes in your elbow and then, all of a sudden, in your shoulder? Is it a dull pain or sharp?"

"It is mostly a deep, dull, constant pain," I answered.

And, *Yes!* I said. It most definitely did jump around! Sometimes from my wrists to my ankles and elbows and even my neck! "My mom and dad used to put me in hot baths," I told him, "and that helped some. Being in the ocean also soothes it, but the pain would never go completely away."

Like Shander, Dr. Phillips began asking me about Lyme disease, whether my family had spent any time in Lyme hotspots like the Hamptons or Martha's Vineyard.

"Nantucket and Bridgehampton," I said.

He asked if I had any other recurring maladies as a child and I told him about the strep throats and headaches. He asked me what doctors had diagnosed me with, and I gave him the rundown.

He asked me if I'd been tested for Lyme disease.

"Three or four times," I said. "The tests came back negative, inconclusive, or borderline."

Dr. Phillips shook his head slightly at my response, or at least that's how it seems in my memory. I adjusted myself for the fifth time within the seven minutes of sitting on his itchy chair. I was getting a hot flash. I started peeling off layers from a light sweater, to a cotton tee, and down to a tank top. I felt embarrassed at the outfit change but he didn't seem to notice.

He led me into his examination room down the hall and left the room so I could undress and put on the cloth medical robe that was folded on the brown fake-leather examining table with the loud white paper. I struggled to get on top of the exam table and made so much noise that the doctor came in and helped me up.

When I looked down at my feet I saw I had put on a pair of mismatched socks: one a green and white reindeer sock, the other with pink and red polka dots. I wiggled my feet like a five-year-old and swayed back and forth; nerves I suppose. The doctor took my blood pressure and temperature and gave me an eye exam, which proved tricky that day. After all, I had missed several road signs on the trip to his office due to my vision going in and out of focus. The doctor scrutinized every joint to see how it functioned. When he got to my hips and knees, I winced in discomfort.

After the exam he led me to a sterile and brightly lit lab, and there he drew my blood. "I am going to use a butterfly needle so it doesn't hurt as much," the doctor said.

I don't know about you, but I don't know why anyone would use the words *butterfly* and *needle* in the same sentence.

Call me crazy, but I don't like anyone taking my blood—even a doctor. When it happens, I tend to get chatty to keep my mind off it. I usually like to ask their astrology sign, or if they have children. So while he drew the blood, I found out that he was single without children and liked to go fishing and camping.

"Ah," I said, "now the shorts make sense."

All told, he took a couple of pints of blood. A couple of pints!

When Dr. Phillips took off the tourniquet and quickly slid the needle out of my arm, he gave me a little paper cup of juice for my blood sugar. I raised the cup in a toast to him and slurped it down. He told me it would take a week or so to analyze the blood.

Dr. Phillips, as it turned out, was as much scientist as doctor. A graduate of the Yale School of Medicine, he researched the microbiology and immunology of *Borrelia burgdorferi,* the Lyme bacteria, for years before he opened his own practice, which, by the way, was booked about as solid as a chic Manhattan restaurant.

Practically bloodless, I somehow managed to crawl back into my car happy that he left me with enough of the stuff to make it home. I'm joking, of course, but it felt like that. On the way, my mind started to swirl with the *What ifs?* What if he couldn't find anything? What if all of the symptoms had been in my head or made up for the past eleven-odd years? What if I was perfectly fine? These thoughts frightened me more than anything. If the blood work was okay, then I was truly crazy, and maybe the worst hypochondriac who ever lived.

I'd have to wait and see—and wait I did. I went about my life, going to Best & Company during the day and to diners and Balder-dash games at night. I also went to estate sales on the weekends, collecting cool vintage handbags, scarves, and accessories. My friend Courtney from rehab would come with me. We had the idea to buy a school bus and ride around the country selling our unique vintage finds from it.

Finally, about two weeks later, the doctor called and told me I needed to come into the office as soon as possible.

If you had seen me drive to Dr. Phillips's office the next afternoon you would have sworn that someone was chasing me. This time Led Zeppelin blasted from my speakers.

I hurried into the little side-of-the-road-office-house-waiting-room.

When he called me in, Dr. Phillips took out the lab work and looked up at me with an earnest and serious gaze. "You've had Lyme disease lying dormant in your body for about eleven years or so," he began.

It was one of those moments, and there weren't many of them in my life, when I didn't know what to say. I mean, how are you supposed to respond to that kind of news? On one hand I felt validated that he had found Lyme: It answered a lot a questions, but it also meant that I had Lyme! So what do you say? "Oh fuck!" or "Oh great!" or "Oh fucking great!" perhaps?

And what was this bit about it being dormant? It certainly didn't feel as if it was dormant. I would come to find that most people who work in the field believe that the infection caused by chronic Lyme disease is never totally eradicated. The pathogen forms persisters, or dormant forms, that can rest in human tissue and survive indefinitely. The infection then can be responsible for symptoms either through direct infection or by pushing the immune system into a kind of overdrive that creates an autoimmune or hyperinflammatory state, much like lupus or rheumatoid arthritis.[11] Someone had to tell me that, of course, and that conversation wouldn't happen until many years later. Back in Dr. Phillips's office, I just wanted to know why I felt like crap.

"I also found a co-infection called babesiosis," the doctor said. "The tick that bit you was carrying both. I am going to put you on a course of medication and antibiotics that will prove that this diagnosis is accurate. I know that your other blood work in the past was inconclusive. When your symptoms flare up, it will be proof that you indeed have these bacteria in your body. But I have to warn you, you will feel a lot worse at first. This is called a Herxheimer reaction."

"Fucking great!"

twenty

BRAIN FOG, HERXING, AND DON HILL'S

"A prolonged illness associated with Lyme disease in some patients is more widespread and serious than previously understood."
—Johns Hopkins Bloomberg School of Public Health

When I got home from Dr. Phillips's office, I was drained and overwhelmed. I was tremendously relieved that I really had a tangible proper diagnosis! I felt like I had won the lottery or something. I know that sounds strange, but think about it. If you have a mysterious illness that you know is there, damaging many parts of your body and life, and a doctor scientifically sees in your blood that there is actually something going on, you feel relieved. I left happy, and arrived home a little freaked out. I told my parents the news and they were also relieved and happy that I was in good hands, and finally, *finally* had some answers!

Now I was left with reality, and a treatment that I had consciously decided to tackle on my own. I don't know if that was a wise choice this early on in the game. I thought that I would have to take one long-term course of antibiotics and that was it—I would be freed from all of the annoying things my body had been dealing with for so many years. How wrong I was.

At home, I stared at the three prescription drug bags I had picked up from our local pharmacy. I was so proud when I walked into the pharmacy to fetch the medication that I thought would be the answers to all of my problems. I had medication that I didn't know how to take, four different types of antibiotic and antimalarial medications with a dense packet of warnings and instructions. Trying to figure out how to set the clock on my DVD player sent me into a spin, so you can imagine what the lengthy, dense manuals for several different medications would do. It felt so complicated.

One of the medications I couldn't take with dairy; another I needed to take separately from the other, and on an empty stomach; with one I'd have to avoid the sun, and so on. And no one had explained the acidophilus, the "friendly bacteria" that I had to ingest to counteract all the harm the harsh antibiotics were causing. Why was it "friendly"? Did that mean the other bacteria in my body were mean or bitchy? Let's put the nice guys back in there—the last thing we want is a bunch of moody bacteria running around. I was afraid to call Dr. Phillips's office because I knew how busy he was. I was unfamiliar with making calls to doctors when you have a question about medication. Dr. Shander was answering some questions for me when she could, but I was so young, so naïve, and immature. I just pondered and did as I was told. I was very relieved and grateful to have a doctor get to the bottom of what was wrong, and bring a real solution to my physical issues. I didn't want to seem like I was questioning anything, but I was determined to get started, even though I was overwhelmed, scared, and confused.

I had other questions: Apparently acidophilus must be refrigerated. But what if you're traveling? What if you never have an empty stomach because you need to keep it full to prevent nausea? What do you do then—take it when you wake up in the middle of the night with the sweaty sheets, insomnia, and nightmares? I failed to take consistent doses of acidophilus at the correct times just because I was overwhelmed by the complexity. The simplest things were too much for me to handle, even a simple task of taking a probiotic in between meals. I later became obsessed with probiotics because I didn't have a choice. Although the treatment seemed overwhelming and frustrating I was grateful for the diagnosis and believed I was finally on a path to health.

I found out from Phillips that babesiosis (pronounced buh-bee-zee-O-sis) is a cousin of malaria and the cause of the night sweats, headache, and fevers I was experiencing. He told me that Lyme disease or babesia affects the body and mind in ways that are hard to believe, such as getting a fever at the same time every day, or getting a headache at the same time, feeling tired but not being able to sleep at night, having no appetite, having trouble remembering where you are going when you are driving, and other forms of memory loss. You can also develop a phobia of the cold.

His symptom list wasn't hard for me to believe because I had nearly every one of them!

Lyme disease is caused by spirochetes, bacteria, he said, that take on different shapes and hide in the middle of the cell walls and mitochondria. They form a membrane that is very difficult to break. Once they have been in your body untreated over time, and eleven years is quite a long time, they become stubborn and they multiply. Though he nearly lost me at *spirochetes* and *mitochondria,* I certainly knew what he meant by *stubborn.*

Phillips had warned me that though he'd found dormant Lyme in me, the only way to know that it was actively affecting me was to take the antibiotics. He also warned me about the Herxheimer reaction which gets its name from Karl Herxheimer, who, along with Adolf Jarisch, studied this reaction to antibiotics; they published their findings in 1895 and 1902.[12]

Want to take a guess at what a Herxheimer reaction is? You know how some people get a little sick after they've taken a flu shot? Well, a Herxheimer reaction, colloquially known as "herxing," is something like that, only about a million times worse. In other words, if I took the meds Phillips gave me and had active Lyme disease, I was going to get very, very sick before I got any better.

It took me a day or two to build up the courage, but I finally got on the antibiotic regime a couple of days later. It would be an understatement to say that the meds made me feel like shit. I felt like tractor-trailers-had-run-me-over-in-the-middle-of-a-desert shit. My body felt as if I hadn't slept for three days straight.

I was miserable, more miserable than ever before. More miserable than when I went into the ER several times with Charlie in Florida. More miserable than when I was in the Fellini hospital in Austria. There was no painkilling option, either. I wasn't supposed to take Valium, or smoke weed to block the pain and nausea. I had no option but to fight and suffer through. And that's what I did. I put on a brave face when I walked downstairs, but I am sure that members of my family thought I looked like death. "Are you sure you want to keep doing this?" they asked. "Are you certain you are on the right treatments? Is it supposed to make you this sick?" they wondered.

I literally had to visualize a real army inside my body, invading the hidden spirochetes inside the mitochondria. Dissolving and nuking the thick barriers of film that had formed around the bacteria. The only issue here was that the bacteria in my body were more intelligent and cheekier than the army I sent in.

This is the short list of things that might happen to you when you're herxing: fatigue, joint or muscle pain, skin rashes, photosensitivity, irritability, paresthesia (prickling, tingling, etc.), dizziness, sleep disturbances, asthenia (loss of strength), muscle cramps, night sweats, hypertension, hypotension, headaches (especially migraines), and swollen glands. Also heavy perspiration, metallic taste in mouth, chills, nausea, bloating, constipation or diarrhea, low-grade fever, heart palpitations, tachycardia, facial palsy, tinnitus, mental confusion, uncoordinated movement, pruritus (itching), bone pain, flulike syndrome, conjunctivitis, and throat swelling.[13]

It really makes you want to wave your hands in the air and cheer "Hooray!" doesn't it? Can't walk? Great! Can't sleep? Even better! Have a fever every evening for four hours? Gold star! Can't remember how to drive? Well done! Losing your hair? Sexy! Feel like you've been beaten with a baseball bat every time you get out of the shower? Awesome! Can't put lotion on your legs because the skin and muscles are too sensitive? You're doing great!

Feel like you're dying?

Wonderful, just wonderful.

The only good news was the severe version of the notorious "Herxheimer" that I went through indeed proved that I had Lyme disease. And that was a relief. It was a major validation. I was *not* a faker, or a complainer, or a baby. I was actually a brave warrioress who had been fighting through this thing for many years. Now I had proof.

Now, as you might imagine, trying to function like a normal human being while herxing can be a bit tricky, especially when doing things that require you to be awake. I would visit friends and ask to lie down on their couch as soon as I walked in the door or, hell, I even rested on those window seats at cafés just to get four minutes of shut-eye. I am a ball of a contradiction at times. On the one hand, all I could do was sleep and be in bed. But as soon as I had a teeny droplet of energy, I would show myself that I wasn't weak, that I wasn't going to let this disease get the best of me. I had to prove to myself that I still had a life beyond the depressing sheets of my bed. I also knew that visiting Shander and getting biweekly therapy was going to save me from these dark trenches. So, as my mother would say, I bucked up and I went. One time I was so Lyme-y that I fell asleep on Dr. Shander's living room couch and woke up in her house the next morning. She left me a little note on purple paper in purple ink that I found when I woke up: "Good morning, Beautiful. I didn't have the heart to wake you up. You seemed like you needed to sleep and you looked so peaceful. I had to run to see patients at Silver Hill. Help yourself to some tea. Love, Dr. S."

Taking showers proved too painful for my muscles and skin, which were now throbbing and crawling with pain. The water pressure had to be that of a trickle because of my weak and sensitive muscles. Getting out of the shower and drying myself off with a towel, or putting on my daily dose of body moisturizer, was a task I dreaded greatly. It felt like I was severely bruised all over, and that someone had exfoliated my skin with sandpaper for one hour straight. I quickly took to air drying and not caring about having dry skin in the winter.

To sum up this period of my life, I would have to say it went something like this: sleep, no sleep, torture, agony, boredom, frustration, different doctors, my loving and supporting friends, making art in the middle of the night, playing solitaire, sobriety meetings, keeping the cereal industry going with my thrice-daily consumption, and all the while, puffing away on Marlboro Lights and drinking Diet Coke.

I had to stop working at my mom's company. I felt like a four-year-old, and the menial tasks like sorting the swatches were over-whelming me. My brain was like a fog machine in a Steven Meisel shoot. Did I explain the brain fog? It feels like you have done about six bong hits consecutively and are trying to speak at a White House press conference.

I don't know how people work during a Herxheimer, or toler-ate heavy antibiotics while fighting a disease. All I could do was lie in bed, or on a couch, or in a bathtub, or on a floor, or on a window seat, or in the backseat of a car, or . . . you get it, right? When friends would come to visit me it was like they were visiting John and Yoko during a bed-in, except I didn't have a John. My brother Richard, who was living at my dad's at the time, kept me company when he wasn't in school and I beaded jewelry, cut and sewed old T-shirts, sketched, and did anything creative one can do from a bed. A few times I dragged myself into my art studio. There I used my brain fog as a way to trick myself into feeling stoned so I could access that cre-ative "zone" and release myself onto a canvas.

I hadn't smoked a joint since I left Barrett House. Shander told me that pot wasn't good for Lyme patients. "You need a powerful immune system that will fight for you," she said. "The minute you give marijuana to your ranks you have very lazy soldiers. They don't even know which way the war is." Back before my diagnosis, the pot had helped with the nausea and made me feel less anxious, but I took her word for it and left it alone. In front of the canvas, I didn't know what I was painting and I didn't care. I wasn't going to let any-one see the work. I just needed to do it so I knew I could.

After three or four months of this, ahem. . . . Let me write that again in case you didn't catch it the first time, after *three or four months* of herxing, I started to feel a little better. I was able to get out of bed for lengths of time and I could accomplish one or two things a day.

By the fall of 2004, I started to feel more like myself. My dad had moved into an apartment on Mercer Street in SoHo and I spent at least half my time in the city with him. Courtney and I didn't buy the school bus but we did clean out my father's gym in his house in Connecticut and set up appointment-only trunk shows. We called our company All the Tea in China.

One of the things about coming off months of herxing and starting to feel better is you have a surge of energy and a need to make up for all the time you lost in bed.

I decided that I wanted to go to acting school and move toward the creative work that I'd always been passionate about. I applied to Stella Adler Studio of Acting, was accepted into the program, and found my own little apartment a block away from the studio. Courtney helped me move into it.

I spent about a year studying at Stella Adler, met cool people, did fun acting scenes, and loved hanging out with weird theater people. The experience reminded me of *Abby's Song* and that wonderful time in my life.

After Stella Adler, I enrolled at HB Studios, where I continued my acting studies. Around that time, we bought an apartment in SoHo on Greenwich Street. I came down with the flu. The doormen and maintenance man took turns going to the deli to buy me Gatorade and ginger ale because I was too weak to get out of bed. I finally felt well enough to staple sarongs and scarves together and tacked them over the windows with thumbtacks to create temporary curtains.

Right next to the apartment, however, was Don Hill's, the club where Uncle Andy and Billy performed, and where we had Billy's memorial. Don Hill himself was always sitting outside his club on a bar stool. A waify fellow with a long, gray ponytail, he was always dressed in denim and Native American jewelry. After I moved in next door, Uncle Andy told Don to look after me while I lived in the neighborhood. He did, too, but only from his perch on the bar stool.

I'd started a tradition of having Sunday dinner at my apartment with friends and family and anyone else who was around. For me growing up, Sundays were always dull and dismal, so when I was on my own, I decided I was going to make it something to look forward to. The dinners usually consisted of eight or ten people from the various creative worlds I inhabited. I would cook my favorite meals; usually roasted chicken with tons of roasted vegetables, or a rosemary lamb roast. It was always a lot of fun. I've always been a good cook; it just comes naturally. I invited Don to come, more than once, but I think he was too shy.

Years later, Don's club would provide the setting for a big moment in my life.

twenty-one

DAD, LIGHT
THE NAG CHAMPA

"Undisturbed calmness of mind is attained by cultivating friendliness toward the happy, compassion for the unhappy, delight in the virtuous, and indifference toward the wicked."
—Patañjali, *The Yoga Sutras of Patañjali*

Doctor number three.

Back when I was fifteen years old and living with my dad on the Upper West Side, my loving father sought out a way to save both of us. He had no idea why his marriage had just ended and I had no idea why I had chronic joint pain. Through his efforts he hoped he would be spared a dark depression and turning into a vacuous playboy, and I would be rescued from chronic physical agony on a daily basis and also the sadness that comes with being the eldest child of divorcing parents.

So how did he do it?

He called Yoga Joe.

Joe was an Ashtanga yogi who happened to be a Tommy Hilfiger fit model. A fit model is a guy or girl whose measurements are so precise that designers are able to fit the sizes of the clothes that they make according to this person's body. Then you work up and down in inches from the size of the fit model to make the various sizes, which is called grading.

Strikingly handsome, Joe looked like a version of Brad Pitt, but he was an odd fellow and when he spoke you had to wonder if he'd been doing yoga and meditating for too long. Joe really liked women. He really liked a lot of women. He never seemed able to control the inappropriate comment about rear ends, mine included. But he was a great teacher for us. He was truly dedicated to his yoga practice and very strict. My dad and I needed someone to keep us in line, because he and I tend to giggle and act immaturely.

Sanskrit for "eight limbs," Ashtanga is made up of eight components: Yama: moral codes; Niyama: self-purification and study; Asana: posture; Pranayama: breath control; Pratyahar: withdrawing of the mind from the senses; Dharana: concentration; Dhyana: deep meditation; and Samadhi: union with the object of meditation.

Joe taught us every pose in the Ashtanga series and pushed us to improve upon every single one of them. No slacking under Yoga Joe's watch.

My dad would wake me up every morning at six o'clock with the Sting song "Fields of Gold" playing on the stereo. He had a pot of coffee brewing and the Nag Champa incense was lit. It was heaven. We drank a cup of coffee together and welcomed Yoga Joe into the apartment to start our practice at six thirty.

We chanted at the beginning and the end of class. Another stick of incense was lit at the start of class and the smell of the Nag Champa, along with barrels of sweat drenching our mats and the feeling of the warm sun on my face while sitting on a yoga mat, is one of my strongest sense memories, as they would say in acting class.

We became so consistent that I can do the sequence with my eyes closed to this day, although you are technically supposed to keep your eyes open the whole time, according to Yoga Joe.

The yoga practice alleviated my joint pain significantly but certainly not permanently.

It was around this time that I realized that managing my well-being was not an exact science. Sometimes it's just unmanageable. You fall down. You eat things that will cause inflammation because they're covered in frosting and look pretty. You go on a date and oversleep for yoga. You push yourself too hard at work and pay the price with exhaustion the next week. Though I didn't know this then, Lyme recovery is not linear and Lyme sufferers are human. We make bad decisions or no decisions, which might delay recovery, but we must forgive ourselves and keep moving. I have learned that living with long-term Lyme disease, or any autoimmune illness, I suppose, means managing it through healthy diet, and sleep. A reduction of stress is key, too, but nearly impossible for most. I wish there was one thing I could do or take, not keeping a million balls in the air to feel well. It is a full-time job to stay healthy. Sometimes it is easy to just want to let loose and say, Fuck it, I am going to have a piece of pizza and a beer. Just know that the next day, you will have to suffer through the consequences.

We're never completely cured, but we find a life that's manageable.

By 2005, I'd exhausted all of the treatments that Dr. Phillips had me on, including tetracycline, an oral antibiotic. When I took that stuff, I had to avoid the sun, threw up a lot, had diarrhea, and the slightest task would leave me completely exhausted. I remember one day when I was on the tetracycline I nearly collapsed on the stairs. It was so scary. I felt lightheaded several times throughout the day, but when it happened as I was trying to walk to bed, I was very grateful I had a friend there to help me up and just sit with me on the stairs for a good thirty minutes.

The tetracycline episode convinced me that I needed to try another approach and I went to Shander again to ask her to recommend another doctor.

Please don't get the wrong idea. I thought Dr. Phillips was an amazing doctor and he helped me a great deal; I was just so sick of being sick from the medicine. I would come to find out that most of the medical treatment for Lyme is no picnic. Back then, however, I thought there must be an easier way.

Though he hadn't yet written *Why Can't I Get Better? Solving the Mystery of Lyme & Chronic Disease,* his bestselling and seminal book, Dr. Richard Horowitz (doctor No. 3) was already one of the foremost Lyme experts in the country. It was nearly impossible to get an appointment with him. I thought I had better use my resources and have my dad make the appointment and accompany me. If there was one time in my life I was going to drop my own name, it was now.

I knew I was going to like Dr. Horowitz as soon as I entered his waiting room. A very large space, it was filled with crystals and old statues of Buddhist and Hindu origin, a big aquarium, and nature magazines. I thought I'd found another kindred spirit, or a Hindu man or Tibetan monk I knew from a past life.

Handsome, and with a scruffy salt-and-pepper beard, Horowitz proved to be pretty good in this life, too. He was funny, kind, open, and didn't question any of the strange symptoms with which I walked into his office. He examined me and took down my medical history. Then he took my blood and reviewed my previous blood tests from

Dr. Phillips, whom he knew. He didn't need much convincing that Lyme disease and the babesia parasite, which is transmitted through the saliva of a tick when it bites a human, were the main culprits in my case.

Where I really connected with him, though, was when we began talking about my interest in ancient forms of spirituality.

It was during that conversation that he told me about the mantra that his guru gave him. Mantras are very private, and I knew that his telling it to me was both an honor and a matter of trust. "Please do not share this with anyone," he said. He told me to chant it twice a day and promised that it would raise my immune system and benefit my overall health. He then asked me if I had some sort of altar or place where I could meditate.

I did. An acquaintance of ours was a carpenter. While I was in high school and beginning my spiritual search, I worked with him to design a hand-carved alcove-altar in my dad's house for my meditation. On it I placed my coral Buddha, my Ganesh, a big bronze Buddha my mother had given me, and other spiritual items. I burned sage to clear the energy, and it held a very special and important place for me. Oh, and of course I had Nag Champa incense constantly burning along with live flowers.

After Horowitz gave me his chant, which was in Sanskrit, I would sit in front of my altar with the paper he'd written it on, reading it out loud over and over.

Seeing Dr. Horowitz marked a turning point in my quest to cure my disease. He was brilliant in blending Eastern and Western disciplines to fight my Lyme. He was also the first Lyme-literate medical practitioner to prescribe a spiritual discipline along with medication. Yes, Dr. Shander was a big proponent of a spiritual path to well-being, but she was my psychiatrist and therapist. Dr. Horowitz was my Lyme doctor and it felt good to have someone treating me for my primary illness who believed that meds alone were not the answer to my problems. I would come to learn that the battle against Lyme is fought on three levels—physical, mental, and spiritual—and all three are equally important. Actually, I think the spiritual part is the most important.

Here's why the spiritual component matters: In chanting the mantra, I had this insight that my battle with Lyme was allowing me to see a thread that had been in my soul all my life. I began, in that moment, to see my true spiritual nature. I found that I am a very open and accepting human. I am grounded in the belief that positive energy attracts positive energy. I have come to find that when I follow my instinct it always leads me in the correct direction. It's strange that a disease can do that but that's what happened. I saw the beliefs, the familial love, art-making, creativity, and the desire to help others all coming together to reveal who I really am. In going within I found peace and strength. I found resolution within my own self. Tapping into this inner strength would be the answer for me. This is not a small thing.

As I battled Lyme, I was becoming who I truly was, and that was the biggest step I took in defeating my illness.

My time with Horowitz wasn't all chants and insights, however. He gave me something called Mepron, a liquid medication given to a lot of AIDS patients as well as people who have contracted malaria. It looks like bright yellow street paint and tastes like sour bubble gum. It's thick and repulsive and lumpy and it turns your tongue bright yellow. The aftertaste needs to be addressed by the scientific community! I used to wash it down with a glass of milk, Lactaid milk in my case. Mepron is not exactly a stroll on the beach. It has a lot of side effects, including mood swings, feeling speedy, and vision impairment.

Dr. H. gave me several other medications as well. To be honest, I was a bit overwhelmed with the very precise routine in which these medications were to be consumed. A friend I'd met in a twelve-step meeting helped me make a schedule and thank God she did, or I would have been lost.

With the meds, however, I knew another Herxheimer was on the horizon, and even though I knew I would feel better afterward, I was scared.

It is tremendously difficult to endure the highs and lows of Lyme disease. I would feel better on antibiotics, live my life and work, then crash a couple of months later and have to go back on antibiotics and stay in bed for long periods of time. The number of Lyme relapses is impossible for me to count. I felt so disappointed in the world and myself when I began to feel the symptoms creep up again, and that's what happened to me after I saw Horowitz for a while.

It was easy to get frustrated and I did, not with Dr. Horowitz, but by having to take all the meds and then go through yet another reaction to the antibiotics. I wanted to be done, cured, and better. I didn't want to have to fight all the time and the routine was tiring.

Dr. Horowitz's office was in Hyde Park, New York, which is halfway between New York City and Albany, and at least an hour and a half from Greenwich, even considering how I drive. A trip to the grocery store would leave me exhausted, never mind spending three hours in the car commuting to my doctor's office once or twice a week. What's more, his program was very intense, and my visits with him lasted a couple of hours. Perhaps it was too intense for me, or perhaps I was just looking for an excuse to stop going.

I saw Dr. Horowitz for nine months, and during that time I took an enormous quantity of medicine. My father and I would walk out of the doctor's office with barrels of antibiotics and herbs!

As I got better, though, taking the whole day for a doctor's appointment seemed even more inconvenient than all the meds I had to take. It was certainly inconvenient for Dad, who always came along despite his busy schedule. Eventually I heard about a Lyme doctor whose office was just down the street from my mom's house. I decided to look into seeing him. Besides, thanks to Dr. Horowitz, I really started to feel pretty good.

One of the most deceptive elements of Lyme disease, however, is that when you start to feel better you think it's forever.

twenty-two
STRAIGHT TO THE HEART

*"Approximately 10 percent to 15 percent of people
who are treated for medically documented Lyme disease
develop persistent or recurrent symptoms of fatigue,
musculoskeletal pain and cognitive complaints."*
—New York Times

For the most part, I didn't involve my mother with my doctors' visits and the Lyme carousel I was on. She was still raising children (my two younger sisters) and running a company. She was also then in a weird place because of her separation with my dad.

But I love my mother dearly. She is a truly amazing and insightful woman. Being around my mom is like being around a fairy child, a female Peter Pan, if you will.

Mom has a way about her. You cannot resist her or her charming demands.

I think I was about eleven years old when my mother strongly suggested that we take a trip to Lourdes, France. My mother is very spiritual, as I have explained, and her spirituality covers a large spectrum. When my mother told Sister Sheehan (the flying nun who raced me to the ER when I had the noodle stuck up my nose) that we were going to Lourdes, Sister Sheehan exclaimed, "No! You can't do that! You must be a part of a pilgrimage!" My mother responded with a quiet, confident answer, "Well then, I suppose it is in God's hands." And it was. Apparently, Mother Mary had appeared in Lourdes about eighteen times. It is a healing place, and there is a hospital for the mentally and physically disabled there. Somehow, my clever mom managed to get us a volunteering gig at the hospital.

So, one very hot summer day, off we went on this pilgrimage to France.

Lourdes is in the foothills of the Pyrenees Mountains. We were driven up a set of windy roads that led to a small classic French town with a church in the center. We stayed in a hostel run by a plump, homely, older woman who showed us to our little room. The accommodation included two small, single beds clad in artichoke-colored blankets, a shower fit for Tinker Bell, and a tiny toilet. The sink stood like a birdbath in the middle of the room away from the toilet or shower. Very European. My mother wasn't impressed. She took one look at the room and let out a little gasp, after which she held her breath with her cheeks as large as balloons.

"Well," she said with an exhale, "at least the color story in here is mustard," which, according to Mom, is "very chic, very Lanvin."

I plopped on the little bed and opened a book I was reading. Although I can't recall the title, I do remember is was a bit racy for my age. The heroine of the story had married a mean man who "wouldn't stop bothering her on their honeymoon," events that would leave her in pain afterward. I really didn't understand it at first, but when I finally got what they were talking about I felt embarrassed and hid the book from my mom—but I kept reading when she wasn't looking.

Anyhow, the next day, after a few bland meals in our room, we ventured into the hospital, where two small, thin older nuns in interesting blue habits met us. They showed us around the hospital and in broken English explained what our daily duties and hours would be. The head nun called me "Une Petite," aka "Little One." Our job was to change soiled and wet sheets on the patients' beds. Distracted, I tried very hard to not to show the shock I was experiencing. I think I might have even begun to cry a little when I saw the all the people in wheelchairs, most of whom seemingly had little brain activity at all.

Still, my mom and I stayed chipper and chatty with everyone who worked there and especially with those poor residents of the hospital. Why not bring a little warmth and human interaction into their lives?

"Madam, Une Petite," the old head nun began, "s'il vous plait, you may no speak wiz za patients."

Mom and I started to giggle like Lucy and Ethel from *I Love Lucy*. Not a smart move.

"I am afraid I weel af to move you and Une Petite to za kitchen," said the nun, "for za cooking of za lunch an dinner."

Which sounded just fine to me. Cooking in a French kitchen or changing soiled sheets? Not really a toss-up, except that the nun didn't mean that we would be cooking anything. What she meant to say was that we were going to clean off the tables and then wash the dirty dishes.

So off Lucy and Ethel went to zee kitchen.

In between our shifts, my mom and I would walk down the hill past the church with the little steeple and into the heavily flooded tourist trap call Lourdes. I don't mean any disrespect, but come on! The lines to see where Mary appeared were insane, like Disney World in July. To touch the holy water was the ultimate goal. In line to do so, my mom was by turns chatty and then arguing with people she thought were cutting the line or brushing up against her. The sights around me moved me, though. I saw everyone from terminal cancer patients to disabled children and adults in wheelchairs, similar to the patients at the hospital, and everyone in between. I had the thought that maybe the water could help me, too, but I quickly dispelled it. My aches and joint pains seemed small compared to the problems of the people in line with us. When I did, eventually, get my hands on the water, I prayed for my siblings, my family, and the people I'd seen in the hospital and in line. But I snuck a little prayer in there for myself at the end, just in case.

My mother scheduled a private hands-on healing *in* the holy water for the next day. That evening I got the flu with a high fever (how's that for healing waters?) and was too sick to get out of the bed to witness my mother waiting in line again, putting on a swimsuit to get into water that millions of other people had been in, and then have some random person in a bathing suit touching her.

Instead I stayed in bed, sick, reading my racy book.

When Mom came back, though, she did look different: vulnerable and serene. She told me how the holy blessing in the water allowed one intention and all she prayed for was her children.

It was beautiful and sweet.

As with some of the other doctors I had seen, for example Shander and Phillips, Dr. Kenneth Liegner's office was in his home (doctor No. 4). I remember his waiting room as being small, cold, and filled with environmental and political magazines. Though his waiting room was a bit nondescript, his personal office looked as if it belonged to a Lyme hoarder. Piles and piles of medical books and manila folders filled every available space. He knew so much about the disease, when he explained it to Dad and me it was like taking a crash college course. Every doctor explains Lyme disease in a different type of way, or maybe I just pay attention at different parts, but the way he explained things to me all made a lot of sense. He was not afraid to dive into scientific depth, in fear of patients not being able to comprehend, but my father and I understood a lot of it in ways that we never had before. On his walls hung the usual array of diplomas, but what caught my eye was the Hippocratic Oath in various languages, beautifully framed. When I asked him to explain to me what one meant, he did so with such passion it made me feel safe that I was in his care.

I liked Dr. Liegner a lot, though he didn't have Horowitz's bedside manner. In fact, he seemed a little preoccupied but in a good way, as if he was always thinking about me and my case. I'd tell him a joke and he'd chuckle a minute later because he was thinking about something like how thick the film was around the spirochetes hibernating in my cells' mitochondria. He also always looked tired, as if he'd been up all night studying my file, and he seemed a bit nervous when he was explaining, as if he knew how fragile Lyme patients are.

One day, after I'd been seeing him awhile, he asked my dad and me if we would be willing to support the Time for Lyme charity gala, which was approaching. He was very nervous about asking us. He kept saying things like "The only reason I am asking you is because it will help a lot of people" and "The woman who founded this is a good woman who, along with her children, battle this horrible disease." He was a very humble man.

"Of course," my dad said before the doctor was halfway through his pitch. "We'll do whatever we can to help."

It's funny how things work out. Time for Lyme turned into Lyme Research Alliance and became a part of Global Lyme Alliance. GLA is one of the most influential organizations in the world in the fight against Lyme and one I'm happy to be part of today.

Dr. Liegner believed in a very aggressive approach to fighting Lyme disease, including the long-term use of a peripherally inserted central catheter (PICC) line for IV antibiotics. For seven months I had a tube sticking out of my arm that was connected to my heart.

Let me say again: *It was in my heart!*

What perhaps frightened me the most, however, was the process of inserting the tube, which involves using a wire as a guideline that they would thread through my arm and into my heart. Again, that was *into my heart!*

At first, Dr. Liegner attempted to insert the PICC line himself, in his office with topical Novocain. The wails that flew out of me were heard in the waiting room. There, pacing back and forth in her ballerina flats with grosgrain bows, my mother became undone at a doctor's thinking it would be relatively painless to insert a tube through an incision in her daughter's arm and into her daughter's heart without first putting her under. Mom demanded the attention of the doctor immediately. "Who would do such a thing?!" she exclaimed. "We are taking you to a hospital to do this procedure, Alexandria. I insist."

I am not faulting Dr. Liegner. Undoubtedly he has successfully inserted countless PICC lines with little difficulty, but when it comes to people sticking sharp things into me and then threading a tube through the hole into *my heart,* I'm not your average patient.

I was relieved at the state of my mother's parenting skills. I needed a mama bear. I think the doctor was happy to schedule the procedure at the local hospital in Westchester, and my mother drove me to the appointment three days later. When we got to the waiting area and filled out all the documents, I felt as if I had written a small book. Though the prospect of the PICC line was daunting, a Valium and some numbing cream had me singing to a Beatles' song on my headphones. "Here comes the sun, little darling, here comes the sun, and I say . . ." And before you knew it, the tube was fed through a vein in my arm and was implanted into my heart. "It's all right . . ."

We had a nurse come every morning and every afternoon to administer the IV antibiotics. I was living at my dad's house. The nurses who came were very sweet. The morning nurse came at seven and when she started the drip, I would fall back asleep and wake up to a sudden wave of nausea. It was like my sleeping body knew that some strange foreign substance was running through my veins, and it wanted it to stop. I was prescribed a strong antinausea medication to help with this.

The first attempt with a certain antibiotic almost turned lethal. My whole body shook uncontrollably. A close friend, Dan, thought I was having a seizure (I wasn't but I was close) and rushed me to the emergency room. I took a few days off before trying a new antibiotic.

Medication on medication on medication.

Before I went on the PICC line, I'd spent weeks planting and cultivating a garden in my father's yard. It was filled with herbs, veggies, and flowers. I loved feeling the earth in my hands and the sun on my back. About three weeks into the IV treatment those moments in the garden seemed like they belonged to another person in another time. In bed I went into a deep depression. My father had met a lovely woman named Dee (they eventually married). One day Dee came up to my room. "Why don't you just go outside and do something?" she said. If I'd had the strength I would have thrown something at her. All I wanted to do was to go outside, but it was difficult for me to make it to the bathroom. In thinking back about that moment, I realize now how representative it is of one of the main difficulty Lyme sufferers face: not being taken seriously, or being accused of exaggerating our suffering. Though the idea that someone would go to such lengths to garner sympathy or attention might seem far-fetched, this reaction people have to Lyme is pretty common—and understandable.

Dee's remark hurt me, but I didn't say anything to her.

Along with being extraordinarily beautiful, Dee is a smart, tough cookie. I was thrilled when she came into my dad's life. She was just what he needed. Though I was upset at Dee's remark, in looking back I can't really blame her. Throughout my illness, and for months at a time, I lived and acted like a normal, healthy girl. Dee saw me travel often to Europe. She saw me being social and happy at weddings and family gatherings and working hard, so why wouldn't she think I was exaggerating? How could I seem so healthy one day and so sick the next? What she didn't see were the days in between, the Lyme flare-ups or the reaction to the meds. The symptoms under the surface, like joint pain, headaches, and confusion, are invisible to the world. Sometimes symptoms of Lyme don't seem unbearable to many people as well. To some, the thought of a headache or a bit of joint pain is no big deal. What they don't understand is that pain is stronger than normal, constant, and nearly every day, on top of a slew of other annoying strange and frustrating things. A little Motrin and fresh air just doesn't do the trick *at all*.

Dee would come to understand, and sometime later, at a Lyme awareness fund-raising dinner, we would have a touching and bonding moment. "I had no idea how much you had to endure," she would tell me that night as she hugged me tenderly. "You are so strong and I'm so incredibly proud of you and you have come so far."

I saw doctor No. 4, Liegner, for three years and for much of the time he had me on oral antibiotics. When I went off the meds, I'd push myself through the winters, trying to prove to everyone around me as well as myself that I was on my way to beating Lyme disease.

I wasn't beating it. Instead, I was losing a little bit more of myself to it every day.

twenty-three

SMELLING LIKE GARLIC
AND LOVING THE HIGH

For stretches under Liegner's care, again in the fall and winter, I'd feel healthy and eager to make up for lost time. I put together art shows, did styling for models in magazines and for a few musical bands, went out every night, and had a great time. I loved meeting new people; I loved working on new projects and pulling clothes for photo shoots. I loved waking up early to go on a set and dress models and come home and paint. I started a little freelance styling gig and my first major client was a Latina pop star who had some hit singles in the United States. This girl was a sweetheart. Her managers? Not so much. Still I worked my butt off for them for three months straight and loved every minute of it. I had my health back and I was ready for whatever life handed me. Finally, I was ready to be a fully healthy functioning adult.

Well, that's not exactly true. I had formed a habit of denying my symptoms and pretending they weren't creeping up on me. I thought

I could *believe* my way out of my disease. I'm all for positive think-ing, but there is a big difference between positive thinking and denial. I would lie to myself when I was exhausted and blame it on work. I couldn't remember things. I was just tired. I would blame my joint pain on walking too much in high heels—I was only twenty-four, for goodness sakes! Still, you can keep the ruse up for only so long. There comes a point when you just have to stop lying to yourself and others.

There also comes a point when you can't lie anymore.

In March 2007 I planned a surprise birthday party for a friend. By the time all the guests had arrived and yelled "Surprise!" I'd crashed on his bed, where I stayed for the entire party. Mind you, I had organized the whole thing, so I was basically the hostess who passed out in the back room while everyone enjoyed the party.

As spring came, I began experiencing severe brain fog, joint pain, and undeniable fatigue. My speech slowed and just about any movement in my joints became painful. I had to walk with a cane a couple of times. All I wanted to wear was loose sweats or men's khakis (a great look for an aspiring stylist!) because the feeling of anything tight on my body was restricting and frankly, painful. I called my father nearly in tears.

"I think the Lyme is back, and I don't know what to do."

My father was adamant about one thing: No rock should ever go unturned. No treatment should be ignored or unexplored.

"We have to try something new."

My parents were scared and maybe more so than ever before. Weren't the treatments working? Hadn't I stayed home three or four summers in a row getting well? What went wrong? Why didn't the powerful army of antibiotics work?

Then one day, as if he were Sherlock Holmes uncovering a clue, my father announced, "Chinese medicine!"

He came home that day all excited, with a lot of information about how effective Chinese medicine and herbs were at helping patients with hepatitis, HIV, and cancer.

"They boost your immune system so much that the spirochetes can't live in the body anymore!" he proclaimed. "This is the most ancient form of medicine in the world! It has to work! And Dr. Horowitz swears by this guy! We have to give him a try."

And so I was off to see to see the extraordinary Dr. Qingcai Zhang. Doctor No. 5.

His office was in a charming house with trellises of wisteria and fountains all around it. It was magical, especially in the springtime.

My mother was impressed.

My dad was very excited.

I was annoyed.

Here I was going to yet another doctor and I knew he would load me up with yet another major treatment program that would require even more effort than the antibiotics.

I was fed up with having to fight this disease once again.

Every time I thought I'd found the right doctor or the right treatment, I'd discover it was just part of the answer or a temporary fix. It becomes even more frustrating as treatments underachieve or fail outright. It's not that the doctors and medicine were bad, it was just that the disease was better, smarter. Sooner or later, every person reaches the same point in their recovery: They give up hope that life will ever be normal again.

I started feeling sorry for myself and thinking, *What is the point of this, anyhow? I am probably going to have to live like this forever, be this fragile sick dumb girl who probably can never be a mother, or a good partner. Who the hell would want to put up with any of this? What man would be able to stand my constant bouts of dry heaving over a toilet, or night sweats, memory loss, and depression? I am destined to have a lonely, lousy life.*

I'd developed a big case of the "fuck-its," but sitting on the pity pot was only going to make me stink.

Dr. Zhang took my pulse and looked at my tongue and my eyes and listened to my heart. He could tell that my body had been through the wringer. My immune system was shot. My body was filled with Lyme bugs, some dead, some alive, hence the reason I felt so Lyme-y.

"We have to clean and boost you," he said.

Dr. Zhang is the preeminent author of *Lyme Disease and Modern Chinese Medicine*, a book on the benefits of Chinese herbs in the fight against autoimmune diseases like Lyme. He's actually a really big deal.

"We must be aggressive," he said. "But you must remain consistent and disciplined."

Consistent and disciplined? *What the heck does he think I've been doing for the last four years of my life?*

We walked out of Dr. Zhang's office with four large paper bags filled with herbs and Chinese medicine and specific instructions on how to consume these magic remedies. I would be putting something from the bags into my mouth about every two to three hours. For all I knew I was going to smell like stale monkey feces.

Thank God I'm single, I thought.

Leaving Zhang's office, my dad sensed how down I was and came up with an idea. "Mustique!" he announced. "It's the healthiest place in the world!"

My mom immediately volunteered to come with me. She was ready to forge through this process with me, her eldest daughter, and put her business aside. My father would look after the other three children (who were in their teens).

My mom packed enough glamorous and fabulous clothes to last both of us for at least two years. I felt like Mrs. Howell on *Gilligan's Island*. (By the way, why did Mrs. Howell have all of those fabulous outfit changes if she was only going on a three-hour tour? As a stylist, I loved that the costume guy ignored that fact and just dressed her to the nines any chance he could.)

Anyway, I hobbled onto the plane with my cane, in my baggy men's paint-stained khakis, bleary and teary, and slept the whole way. I left everything and everyone behind except my canvases, paints, and brushes. I must admit, I was excited to go on this adventure with my mom. I'd hoped we were embarking on something that would make us both stronger.

On our first day in Mustique, both Mom and I started on the herbs (Mom was taking them as a show a support and because they are supposed to be good for you even if you're not suffering from Lyme) and I immediately lost any fear of being attacked by a vampire. The Zhang treatment involved ingesting copious amounts of garlic pills to boost the immune system. Garlic was oozing out of my pores. When my sister Elizabeth came to visit she'd walk by me and hold her nose.

After dinner, I'd play a game of gin rummy with Arlene, a family friend and masseuse. After playing gin, Arlene would give me a massage while my mom would putter around the room putting the knickknacks and throw pillows back the way they were when she and my father were together. We would laugh about the happenings of the day and talk about life. It was lovely.

I was then put to bed, literally. I was in so much physical pain and had such bad headaches that Arlene and my mom would have to help situate me in the bed and usually put warm-water packs under my hips and knees to relax them, along with a cold compress on my head. I still had Mutsy, the stuffed dog my mom's seamstress gave me, and he helped keep my knees from rubbing together. Some nights I was brought to tears from the pain. I didn't want to take painkillers because they barely made a dent. I was afraid of prescription meds because I didn't want to poison my body and form an opiate addiction. Looking back, a painkiller would have saved me from nights of agony.

The shittiest part of it was that I could never stay asleep. I would wake up four times during the night, tossing and turning, and have to hobble to the bathroom to pee. At about four or five in the morning I would finally fall asleep for the last time, then wake up at around ten thirty or eleven, eat breakfast, take the herbs, and then lie down again.

Before lunch I would sometimes try to get in the ocean. On the Caribbean side of the island, the water is a lighter turquois, and on the Atlantic side it's a vibrant light sapphire. The ocean water off Macaroni Beach, called that for its shape and white sand, is practically magnetic with negative ions, which are oxygen atoms charged with extra electrons that are extremely beneficial for health. It feels amazing being in the water off Mustique. I swear to God this island holds magical healing powers—but not necessarily for Lyme sufferers.

Though I was in paradise, my body was getting worse. I knew it had to get worse before it got better and I had to endure yet another Herxheimer flare-up, but this one seemed to be extraordinarily painful.

Somehow, I painted every day and the pieces I made were different than any I'd done before; it came like a stream of sunlight through the storm clouds. That creative burst, and my friends who visited (and Mom, of course), are what kept me from going over the edge.

twenty-four
HEAD, SHOULDERS, KNEES, AND...FINGERNAILS?

"Most medical experts believe that the lingering symptoms are the result of residual damage to tissues and the immune system that occurred during the infection."

—Centers for Disease Control

Along with the doctors who treated me for substantial periods of time, I also saw at least four doctors (there might have been more) for shorter periods and they bear mentioning for a variety of reasons. These are doctors Nos. 6–9.

There was Dr. D'Adamo, in whose office I sat with my video camera because I was having problems remembering, and not only did I want to personally understand his treatments, but I wanted to be able to explain them to others when they asked me about them. Dr. D'Adamo measured every part of my body, from my feet to the width of my fingernails. He measured the circumference of my head and my eyeballs, the length of my fingers. By this analysis he was able to determine my genotype and tailor a diet for me that would help me fight Lyme and find optimal health.

According to D'Adamo, there are six major genotypes, which he called the hunter, the gatherer, the teacher, the explorer, the warrior, and the nomad. I was kind of hoping I'd fall into warrior or nomad category but settled for the explorer with my O-negative blood type. I'd certainly been on a journey exploring different solutions and treatments. I followed his very specific diet to a T. I couldn't eat ham, bacon, eggs, cheeses, beef, and poultry, but I could have lamb, mutton, rabbit, and goose and quail eggs. It was as if I were cooking for Robin Hood and his merry men. There are only so many meals you can make with goose eggs. I do believe in this diet, and still follow it as much as I can to maintain optimal health.

In no order of importance or chronology, the next doctor we'll call "Dr. K." My dad and Dee met me at his office. Dr. K. had a Middle Eastern accent, round, black glasses, and a thin ringlet of a ponytail that fell over the black turtleneck he wore. He sort of reminded me of Steve Jobs but only if Steve Jobs had been cast as the villain in a James Bond movie. I still have the mark on my ass from the penicillin injection Dr. K. gave me. The needle was about the size of a curling iron. At one point during "the procedure," I took out a baguette, which I happened to have in my bag, and bit on it as if it were a stick and he was digging a bullet out of me in an old western.

Though Dr. K. needed to work on his injection technique, he was actually brilliant, but I couldn't handle the protocol of these once-a-week injections. They did nothing that I noticed, anyhow. I am sure someone with a higher tolerance for large needles and penicillin would do well on this treatment, but it was too much for me.

I also went to a doctor whom I won't even merit with a made-up name. He didn't take my blood, thought Lyme doctors were quacks and money-grabbers, and said to me, "You just need to exercise and go on antidepressants." If antidepressants were the answer I would have been cured three years before! Because of depression brought on by my Lyme disease, I had to go on Lexapro in between treatments.

What is even more unbelievable is that this guy worked in Greenwich, Connecticut, which is as close to ground zero of the Lyme epidemic as you can get. It was shocking that a doctor at a hospital in one of the most concentrated areas of Lyme could be so in the dark and dismissive.

My parents also took me to an infectious diseases specialist. He looked at the blood labs and said the titers and bands indicated that I had been exposed to Lyme, but that I was probably just tired from all of the long-term antibiotics. He wanted to put me on glutathione, an antioxidant given to cancer patients (I wasn't a candidate), and said that many Lyme patients just have to put up with symptoms their whole lives because there is no cure for feeling "low-grade shitty all the time." He also said that it didn't make sense that I felt so horrible after every Lyme treatment.

Unfortunately, this doctor isn't alone in his beliefs. Many in the medical community don't think chronic Lyme disease even exists. Even the CDC has trouble acknowledging it. Instead, the government health agency believes that people with Lyme symptoms that last more than six months after an initial antibiotic treatment have post-treatment Lyme disease syndrome, which occurs not because of the *B. burgdorferi* virus itself but because of "residual damage to tissues and the immune system that occurred during the infection," according to the CDC website.[14] I'd be willing to bet that most Lyme sufferers don't give a flying fuck what you want to call it, or who's right and who's wrong. The whole idea here, fellas, is finding a way to cure it.

twenty-five

HAPPY BIRTHDAY, ALLY

"Lyme is the fastest growing vector-borne disease in America."
—Centers for Disease Control[15]

After five months of Chinese herbs, Caribbean Sea water, and Arlene's massages, I felt ready to get back to reality. I never thought I would actually be looking forward to leaving Mustique, but I was.

My mother and I arrived back in New York before the school year was to start and she rented an apartment on the Upper East Side so that Elizabeth could attend high school in the city. My mother did not want to make the same mistake she had made with me, which was letting me attend the Professional Children's School in New York City on my own while living with a father who was so busy, always traveling for business, that he barely slept in the apartment. After I helped my mom move in, I was ready to get my own life moving again.

I knew I was a good designer; how could I not be with the parents I have? My fashion talent is genetic, like my hair color or my Hilfiger mouth. When I decided to start my own clothing collection that fall, I felt as if I was just following a fated path. I called the collection

Alexandria James, after my great-grandfather on my mother's side, the tailor in Little Italy who made the coats for my mother and her siblings when they were children, and I came up with what I thought was a fantastic idea for women's outerwear.

While I was conceptualizing my own line, I began working with a designer named Nary Manivong on his collection—styling, producing, and casting his fashion show. I worked for the Tommy Hilfiger Company for a while that winter as well. I helped with their fashion show, and I worked on an ad campaign in Washington, D.C. As usual, as I started feeling better I went way overboard.

While I was on a photo shoot for a Hilfiger campaign, someone asked me kindly how I had been feeling after such a long battle with Lyme disease. I was twenty-four at the time, and it had been almost six years of yo-yo Lyme treatments. I told her I was feeling much better, but in my heart I knew I was lying. I knew the symptoms were creeping back, but I didn't want to sound like someone who was too unhealthy to do anything with her life. After doing the Zhang treatment and smelling like garlic for five months, I was frustrated and impatient. I didn't understand that natural treatments take a lot longer, and that there is a longer period of feeling not well before you feel better. I was not ready for this type of alternative healing that would ultimately heal me the most in the end. I was fed up with *any* treatment, actually. I don't think my will to live or feel better was that much of a bright flame in my life at that time. I honestly didn't really care whether I withered away or lived life. I lost my will to live, I suppose, that or my body became so ill that it was impossible to go on. That's really the truth. I felt hopeless and ran into a deep depression. Dr. Shander put me back on antidepressants. My body was shutting down yet again and I had to make a real decision: Do I want to live a happy, healthy life, or do I want to die a slow, painful death? The latter was sounding like the inevitable option at this point.

I heard about a German homeopathic doctor in New York who claimed to have a 100 percent cure rate over Lyme. I didn't call him right away. I needed to see someone about the constant nausea I was experiencing again. I used pot to help with it, but I knew I had to get to the bottom of this problem.

The office was on Park Avenue. The doctor promised that I would need just a light anesthesia to do the procedure. The anesthesiologist began counting backward from ten. I was out at eight. I remember waking up and thinking I was at a nightclub sitting in front of a wall of bright lights. I turned to the sixty-something-year-old anesthesiologist and said, "Will you make out with me?"

"Thanks for asking," he answered, "but I'm married."

I fully woke up to the nurses and doctor giggling. When my eyes focused, I realized that the brightly lit "club wall" was actually the ceiling of the procedure room. When I turned to look at the man whom I had asked to make out with me, I realized he was pushing seventy. I think he was flattered.

The doctor said he didn't find anything significant in my stomach but said that I was in need of some prescription probiotics. I walked out of the office feeling like a fraud, again questioning if I was making up the pain in my head.

That same week happened to be my twenty-fifth birthday. A friend of mine, who was pursuing me, wanted to take me on a little birthday getaway. Patrick was kind and safe, and I enjoyed his company, but I had no desire to date him, so naturally I took him up on his offer.

I like living life spontaneously. So I told Patrick not to tell me where he booked us for our weekend getaway. I figured I'd just show up anywhere with a passport and a packed little bag ready for anything.

Patrick happened to be in South Carolina. Our plan was to meet at the airport in the Bahamas. As the plane began its descent, I started feeling very sharp pains in my stomach, which only got worse as the plane landed. I was frightened that my appendix was exploding.

On the way to customs I collapsed. I was just about out of it, on the side of the corridor in the arms of a strange man who, along with his wife, was fanning me. The man happened to be a paramedic from upstate New York. Lucky me! There were a few people crowded around, and I was flushed with embarrassment.

"Miss, are you okay?" the wife asked. They were nice people. They were concerned.

Airport security arrived with one of those industrial orange wheelchairs. The paramedic helped the airport staff hoist me into it. I was so embarrassed, but I really couldn't walk. They carted me off to a medical unit in the airport and a customs officer cleared me. They then transported me into an ambulance. At this point the pain was coming and going and kind of lessening, but it was still there.

I called Patrick. "Hey, I am in an ambulance on my way to the local hospital. I got off the plane and passed out from terrible pains in my stomach."

Patrick had a bit of a southern twang. "What? You're where? Oh my God, are you *okay*? I was just eating conch wondering if you had landed because I hadn't heard from you."

"I gotta go, they are trying to put an IV in my arm. I'll see you at the hospital."

The hospital was really primitive. It smelled like diarrhea and had bloodstains on the floor. After waiting in a hospital bed for about three hours, I explained to them that I felt much better, and that it was probably just bad gas. They released me pretty quickly.

I knew it wasn't gas, but I wasn't about to sit in that place for the evening.

When we arrived at the Atlantis resort, I truly felt better and was looking forward to eating something light and then going to bed. I barely minded the fact that there was only one hotel room for us, even though I had asked Patrick to book two. Nothing was going to happen between us. I was 100 percent sure of that.

We went down to the sushi restaurant to get rice, soup, and ginger ale. In the middle of the meal, Patrick got up to use the restroom. After about twenty-five minutes, I began to wonder what the hell was keeping him. I decided to give him a call.

"Patrick, are you okay? Where are you?"

"I had to come up to the room. I think I have food poisoning. The conch I ate this afternoon must have been bad. I can't keep anything down."

"Oh my goodness, I will be right up."

It took me about ten minutes to walk across the massive grand marble lobby and down the maze of hotel corridors. I finally found the room. Inside, Patrick was curled up on the edge of the bed with a wastebasket next to him. He was sleeping.

I quietly got into my very conservative pajamas and crept into the other side of the bed—that's when the pain hit me again. I went to sit on the toilet, and it only got worse. When I tried to stand up, I couldn't.

This was not good.

I called my dad.

"Dad, I am in Atlantis, of all places. Patrick is passed out with food poisoning, and I am having blinding pain in my stomach. What should I do?"

"Run a hot bath, and try to relax your muscles," Dad said.

"Eat some peanut butter, Ally," my brother Richard chimed in from the peanut gallery. "You probably just need to shit."

"I think I'll try the bath first," I said.

Sitting in the bath didn't do anything. I called my dad back.

"Wake Patrick up," he said decisively. "Tell him to call an ambulance."

Ten minutes later, two paramedics with a gurney and a police officer entered the room. They started interrogating Patrick with questions. I think they thought he was abusing me since I was crying and screaming when he was on the phone calling for help. The poor guy could barely stand up straight, let alone abuse anybody!

We both made it to the hospital in the ambulance and I was going nuts. The pain was worse than ever. I started to get really scared.

They hooked me up to an IV drip of some sort of drug to ease the pain and calm me down. It worked after about forty-five minutes. They also injected my veins with that terrible burning contrast fluid before they put me into the CT scanner.

Three hours later, after sleeping on and off, and hearing a child in the sectional next to me screaming in his own agony, I was glad when the doctor walked in.

"Miss Hilfiger," she began, "you have kidney stones. Two of them."

At this juncture, my poor friend Patrick had to go back to the hotel to tend to his food poisoning. He wanted to stay with me but I told him to go. I was so out of it on painkillers and sleeping on and off, I didn't need a babysitter.

I don't remember how many hours later, the hospital finally released me and I took a taxi back to the Atlantis.

The next day happened to be my birthday. Before we got on the plane to fly back to the States, I was feeling better (the prescription drugs had kicked in), and I wanted to at least see some of the aquariums that Atlantis has to offer. Behind two-inch-thick glass floated an array of magical sea creatures. I so badly wanted to morph into one of those fish and just float and soar past everyone in a blissful state.

Patrick asked if I would ever move to South Carolina, but I politely declined, explaining that New York would always be my home. When I got back to New York, my family had a little birthday dinner and cake waiting at my dad's apartment. By this time I had passed both stones.

The best birthday *ever*!

twenty-six
THE GERMAN PROTOCOL

"As I often tell patients, Lyme disease usually does not kill you the way AIDS does, but it often makes you wish you were dead."
—Dr. Raphael Stricker, a past president of the International Lyme and Associated Diseases Society

I knew in the deepest recesses of my soul that I didn't have many more tries left in me. In a half-dozen years I'd gone to eight Lyme doctors, who had prescribed that many treatments and more. Each time I'd walk out of their offices with my hopes high, and each time I'd see them dashed.

I decided I would give myself one more try to get better. One more try to have the life of which I had always dreamed.

And so the day came when I knew I really had to take charge of this disease—for the last time.

The process would not be easy. I knew there were a lot of moving pieces involved, as well as a lot of needles, which I loathed. I knew there was a lot of discipline and structure to which I needed to adhere. I knew there would be mountains to climb, rivers to forge, and rings of fire to walk through. But I was ready.

A few weeks before my birthday in February 2010, I called the German who claimed to have a 100 percent success rate.

The German's name (doctor No. 10) was Dr. Thomas K. Szulc (pronounced "Schulz"). Sheila Cox, my dad's longtime, trusted assistant, and our longtime friend and makeup artist, Katrina Borgstrom, had told us how terrific Szulc was. I walked into his Manhattan office with my dad. I remember it was Fashion Week, or just after. I wore an oversize vintage Yves Saint Laurent red blouse, waist high, size 24, skinny jeans (that were baggy on me), YSL platform hiking boots, and a faux fur scarf. Though I was in full Fashion Week attire, I was a wreck and in tears. There were rumors on the Internet that I had some sort of eating disorder or cocaine habit, since I had become so thin. It wasn't coke or anorexia that was deteriorating my body. It was Lyme disease.

In the waiting room, Dad and I met a woman named Diane Blanchard, who would become a beacon of hope for me. Along with Debbie Siciliano, Diane was the cofounder of Time for Lyme, which, as I said, became Global Lyme Alliance. They are my very dear friends. I call them my fairy godmothers.

A bit disheveled, the doctor gave me the impression he didn't care much for his outward appearance, but something about him felt magical to me. I remember when he listened to my heart with his stethoscope I began to cry. I became emotional, as if I knew he could heal with his hands. He was quietly compassionate. He explained to my father and me that his treatments could cure the effects of Lyme disease *if* you followed the program exactly. His theory was actually brilliant. He gave the analogy that your body is like a house. If the house has been dirty and toxic for a long while, and if you have exterminated (with antibiotics), then you still have dead bodies lying around and dirt under the rug. "You must scrub your house thoroughly and clean it completely and remove the bodies" (meaning the spirochetes).

"Then we go in and boost the immune system and bring every system back to optimal health."

Made sense. More sense than anything else. I do really well with visuals.

As we were leaving, Diane was in the waiting room with one of her daughters, who was going through a horrible bought of Lyme disease and doing the German protocol. They gave me a lot of faith that this might actually work.

Though I'd talked myself into being a hardened Lyme warrior, and I knew there was no quick fix in treating the disease, my heart still sank when the doctor told me how long I would be on the treatments: For four months, and multiple times a week, I'd have to visit his office. I knew I had to try, but I also knew I couldn't do it alone. I was twenty-five years old and I was too proud to ask for my parents to help me, or move back in with them.

When I was growing up, my cousin Jaimie and I were more like twin sisters than cousins. We are six and a half months apart in age. We used to joke that we were like Patty and Kathy, from *The Patty Duke Show*. We would prank-call the dELiA*s catalog using different voices, like Marisa Tomei's in the film *My Cousin Vinny*: "My boyfriend he doesn't like when I wear poiple. Ya have red?"

As life tends to get in the way of making phone calls and keeping in touch with the ones you love, I hadn't spoken to Jaimie in some months. I was nervous to call her. It was not easy for me to ask people for help, especially the kind of help I now needed. Jaimie and I also have an inside joke that when we are calling someone we pray that instead of them answering we get their answering machine. When the phone was held up to our ears, we used to chant, "Answering machine, answering machine, answering machine!"

This time, I was not chanting. I was praying that she would pick up.

She did.

"Jaimie, the Lyme is back," I said as hard tears began to well in my eyes. "I need to try something new, but it is going to take a lot, and I can't do it by myself."

"I was waiting for your call. You have been on my mind so much lately. I had no idea how much Lyme people suffer until I spoke to a friend who is a nutritionist about it. I didn't realize how much you have really been through. I can't imagine, Ally.

"What do you need me to do?" she asked.

"I need you to come to New York," I said. "I need help getting through these treatments."

"Done." Jaimie was on the plane to New York the next week. She left her whole life in California behind. She put her successful modeling career on hold to help her sick, helpless cousin. Bless her heart forever. She is truly an angel.

When I scheduled my first appointment with Manhattan Advanced Medicine, the home of Dr. Szulc, I was given a "detox diet" that meant no caffeine, no alcohol, no tobacco, no dairy of any kind, no refined sugar, meat only once a week, no wheat, bran, or oats, and nothing processed or packaged. I could eat all the fruit and veggies I wanted. Yikes. No fun. I was told I'd have to stay on the diet for many, many weeks. That sucked. But I had to do it, so I said good-bye everything yummy, gluttonous, and fun.

Jaimie accompanied me to my first doctor's appointment, where we met Lisa, the head nurse. Lisa was in her forties and had gray hair. She was tough, all business, but gave me the impression that she believed in the treatment with all her heart, but only if properly and precisely followed. *Precise* is the operative word.

As it happened, Dr. Szulc wouldn't treat me. He'd resigned his practice to go on a research bender. I was placed in the capable hands of a disciple of Szulc, Dr. David Manganaro, who had worked with him for years and had taken over the practice.

Dr. Manganaro would turn out to be terrific, and though I was somewhat disappointed that Szulc had left, the German's work lived on in Nurse Lisa.

Nurse Lisa was a big proponent of the Szulc method. "Ally, we are going to give you an IV of saline first," she told me. "At the same time, we are going to hook you up to a machine by attaching wristbands to you that will calm your nervous system. Have you been taking all of the homeopathics and vitamins we sent to you last week?"

"Yes, Nurse Lisa," I said. I felt as if I were answering to a nun. Or a German lieutenant. Both are equally frightening.

"You don't have to call me *Nurse* Lisa. Lisa is just fine. This program only works if you follow it completely. Do you understand?"

Jaimie and I answered her in unison. "Yes, Nurse Lisa. I mean Lisa."

First on the agenda was getting an IV drip of saline to flush out my system and hydrate. In the other arm, Lisa drew blood to be sent through a UV light to be "cleared" and put back into me. My wrists were wrapped with Velcro bracelets that were attached to a machine that sent electromagnetic waves into my body to reset my nervous system, which was completely out of whack. They also checked the vibrations in my blood, which told them the amount of anxiety and confusion running through my body. I know this sounds crazy, but those machines worked. I know they did because they showed exactly how I felt.

The cleanse protocol was to go on for about one month, depending on how fast my body detoxed. On a scale of 1 (fine) to 20 (unhealthy), my body was a 22, if that existed. I left the office with brown paper bags filled with more bottles of homeopathic drops as well as supplements. The instructions for the meds were very specific and many of the medicines were from Germany. Some were only to be taken without food. With others, I couldn't use peppermint or spearmint toothpaste or mouthwash, and each dose was to be taken twenty seconds apart from one another. I was to eat an hour before or after taking the remedies. It was all very confusing, and I got hungry just thinking about it.

At home, Jaimie remained an angel. She lined up all the bottles on the countertop with tiny cups in front of each one. She organized the supplements in separate Tupperware containers according to the times of day they were to be taken. The Virgo in her was shining, and the Pisces in me was twirling. I could have never been this organized on my own. I would've tried, but I undoubtedly would've gotten confused and overwhelmed and given up.

Every treatment at Manhattan Advanced Medicine was tailored for my body. I was told that I had to take all of them in the prescribed combination. Taking one of the treatments alone would be unproductive. This is important: Too many Lyme sufferers are using only part of the available arsenal to fight their disease. Just doing vitamins or herbs, or just the IV treatment, or just doing a diet will not cure you. Combining the different treatments to suit your immune system just might.

It's something like the premise behind the drug cocktail they came up with to fight HIV back in the late 1990s. Alone, each antiretroviral did little to help patients, but when given together the combination nearly erased what had been a certain death sentence. Lyme disease in the United States is spreading much quicker than AIDS did in the 1980s—the CDC estimates there are at least 300,000 new cases each year—and though death often came quicker for those early AIDS patients, Lyme kills, too. But it kills by inches and minutes, and while it takes its time trying to kill you, it settles for making your life painfully miserable.

Jaimie stayed with me for four months. Every morning she gently woke me up to take the drops, then let me fall back asleep. Together we would cook a healthy "on diet" breakfast and go to the grocery store. She accompanied me to all the doctor appointments and sat with me through every IV, which took on average about two hours.

Meanwhile, the treatments progressed. Eventually, after my body was detoxed enough, which took a lot longer than anyone was expecting, I was given IV drips of very high levels of vitamin C, homeopathics, and a special form of hydrogen peroxide. These acted as very strong antimicrobials, as they called them. This was the stuff that would kill the Lyme spirochetes, they promised.

I imagined each of the IV drips as a soldier in my army. After the drip was over, I went into a little room where the doctor injected me twenty-five times on my abdomen and back with homeopathics. This was my official ring of fire. This was also one of my worst nightmares. I looked at this grueling process as some sort of initiation process—into what, I did not exactly know. Maybe I needed to go through this to become a stronger warrior, woman, and human being. I refused to be victimized by it. Well, I cried a lot the first few times, and *then* I decided to not become a victim.

Lying on the table with my shirt up, waiting to be injected twenty-five times in my back and stomach, I began to chant: "Ring of fire, ring of fire, ring of fire."

Dr. Shander helped, too. She told me to visualize myself in an ancient Egyptian sarcophagus with priestesses surrounding me, helping me breathe, and chanting healing words.

"What is your only job right now?" she asked.

"To heal," I answered. "My only job right now is to heal my body."

"That's right," she said. "I will remind you every day."

And she did.

It was then, with Shander's help, that I began to realize that my fight against Lyme had begun to change.

When I was going through the Manhattan Advanced Medicine treatments, that relapse had left me more debilitated than before. It was painful and difficult to get out of bed to get dressed for the doctor, or to get into a bath. I was so frustrated and depressed that I physically could not function, let alone mentally function. I called Shander to ask her how to handle this. She told me that I needed to learn how to mother MYSELF. Living alone and being sick is hard. Even though Jaimie was with me, I was battling with my inner child and not allowing myself to take care of her properly. There were times in which I literally needed to talk to myself and tell myself "it's ok, you just need to take a bath, eat something nourishing and lie down to take a nap. I am sorry you are not feeling well, and it's going to be OKAY." I would have to touch my sensitive arm sometimes just as a reminder that I was so fragile. It had been so bruised from the many rounds of IV drips, and my muscles were still very sensitive.

It had been so easy to be discouraged and down on myself at times. I thought I would have to live like this lump of useless human forever. I don't know how, and I cannot tell you why, but I knew deep down that it wasn't true. I knew I had more purpose and much to offer the world. I also knew on some level that I had something very important to accomplish.

It was then I began to step away from being the victim and step toward becoming a healer. A healer for myself. Most real healers have to go through intense physical trials in order to learn how to cure themselves before even thinking about helping others. I'd gone through rings of fire and initiations to begin this last part of my journey, but I knew that I had a long life ahead of me to learn more.

After four months of going to Manhattan Advanced Medicine, I started to feel better. That July, Jaimie and I went to Europe to meet my dad and Dee and their darling little boy, Sebastian, on a boat in the Mediterranean. We had the time of our lives. After the boat trip, Jaimie and I met my sister Elizabeth in Paris. Elizabeth was taking a summer photography course there. As soon as Jaimie and I got off the plane, I insisted that we celebrate with the most exquisite pastries that Paris had to offer. I had been deprived of sweets for too long, and I'd been living on kale, beet and ginger juice, and carob-covered almonds, which I swear made me gain a few extra pounds. Paris and the Mediterranean Sea made me look and feel glowy and fabulous. I felt more like a human, a lady at that. We shopped until we dropped and became addicted to macaroons.

When Jaimie and I returned to New York, I got a call from Nary Manivong, who wanted me to help him with his next collection and fashion show. I told him that I was just coming off a four-month intensive Lyme program and still needed to take it slow. He was very respectful and brought the collection to me, as it came out of the factory, and we worked diligently at my apartment. I made us quinoa-kale salads and roasted veggies.

I received another phone call from Tara Subkoff, a designer friend. She'd started a very popular clothing line years back called Imitation of Christ. It was brilliant. Tara had celebrities of all walks of life modeling for her and wearing her clothes. She held one of her fashion shows at a funeral home on the Lower East Side! When Tara asked if I could help her style her fashion show as well, I agreed. I couldn't pass up the opportunity. I respected the brand, and I liked her.

September rolled around quickly, and by the time Fashion Week came along, I was in full gear again, feeling better than ever. I felt better than I did after any antibiotic treatment. I knew I was on this health wave for the long haul.

This time, I really believed I was cured of Lyme.

I looked great; I was clear, calm, happy, inspired beyond belief, and ready to balance my work-health lifestyle. When Tara asked me to partner with her after we had worked on her show, I didn't have to think twice; we just started a partnership.

We were looking at spaces to open a store and meeting with manufacturers and backers. We went sample shopping and brainstormed on the direction of the new company. My father was going to be our head guide and possible backer. We called him Big T.

After a few weeks of running around, however, I began to get tired. I was still seeing Manganaro and he suggested that I take it slower. I needed to rely on my instincts to do what was best for my body. One of the pluses of battling Lyme disease it that you learn to rely on your gut, and my gut was telling me that a partnership with Tara, as wonderful as she is, was not in my best interest healthwise.

Needless to say, Tara was disappointed when I pulled out of the partnership. What probably made it seem even worse to her is that I quickly decided to open my own clothing company and have Nary come on as partner and head designer. Of Laotian descent, Nary grew up on the streets of Columbus, Ohio. Literally. A Christian mission brought his parents and grandparents to the United States from Laos. One day Nary came home from school to see all of the family's belongings piled up on the sidewalk in front of their home. They'd been evicted, and his parents were nowhere to be found. They'd basically abandoned him, his twin brother, and his little sister.

The children began sleeping in a Dunkin' Donuts, and a park, and then in the local high school. Eventually, the principal of the school caught on and offered some help. Nary put on his own fashion show at the age of seventeen and homeless, after picking up a *Vogue* magazine in the donut shop and teaching himself how to make clothes by reading books on sewing and pattern-making in the public library.

In Nary, I saw another young talented Asian designer like others who had begun to populate the fashion world, people like Phillip Lim and Alexander Wang. From a business perspective, he was a solid choice even if he wasn't as established as Tara.

But the main reason I went with Nary was that the energy just felt more manageable with him. I could take my time making decisions and not feel overwhelmed by having to live up to Tara's great reputation. I felt safer with Nary and knew I could fail and just try again. I knew partnering with him was the healthier move, and I wasn't about to do anything that would risk my health.

As it turned out, I got Nary—or he got me—just in the nick of time. His main backer experienced financial issues and had quit the partnership after Nary's most recent show. When I called him, Nary was in Delaware at a friend's house lamenting his situation. He later told me that the words "I don't know what I am going to do with my life now" were coming out of his mouth as the phone was ringing.

My father was on the phone with me and suggested we work together to start a new line. He told us to get to a fabric store immediately and come up with a concept for our new clothing line. All brands must have a focus, said Big T. I agreed. It makes for a more creative process. I truly believe that the more restrictions you have, whether it be financial, a color palette, a fabric choice, or making the same one design over and over again, the more creative you can become.

Working on the line was a miraculous adventure and challenge. When I was in Paris, I bought a simple black-washed silk shirtdress. It was brilliantly versatile and chic. We decided to base the clothing line around it.

And so we were off. We went to Mood, the fabric purveyor of *Project Runway* fame, to get inspired and buy some fabric for sampling, and started designing. We worked out of my apartment next to Don Hill's at first, and then soon moved into a small studio space on Thirty-Ninth Street in the Garment District, which was attached to our sample maker's factory. Things couldn't have gone any better. Nary and I came up with a name for the brand by putting our initials together, which formed the word *NAHM*. Nary-Alexandria-Hilfiger-Manivong. In Laotian *nahm* means water, and the concept of water is known to be very healthy for a business.

Before our first fashion show in February 2011, Bridget Foley, who is one of the cornerstones of *Women's Wear Daily,* called us. After the interview, we were directed to go downstairs to their photo studio to shoot some pics.

The next day, we woke up to find a photo of Nary and me on the cover of *Women's Wear Daily.* I cried. Nary cried.

I just couldn't believe it.

The Lyme was gone and all my dreams were coming true.

twenty-seven
THE MAN ALL IN BLACK AND A WIDE-BRIMMED HAT

"Love is a gift of one's inner most soul to another so both can be whole."
—BUDDHA

Oh, wait a minute. Something else really big happened that I forgot to tell you about, but to do so I must take us back a couple of months, to December 13, 2010. A friend of mine was curating an art show in the Meatpacking District, and another friend, Francesco, was deejaying the event. They invited me to the show, which was on a Saturday evening.

At the time I had a housekeeper named Iris who would come to my apartment on Saturdays. I was still trying to master this whole work-health balancing act, and my Saturdays were usually spent in bed recharging my battery. Iris was always bugging me about being single and working all the time or resting in bed. "Get out and have some fun, Miss Ally," she would plead. "Have a man in your bed, it will make you happy and your life full."

Basically what Iris was telling me was that in order to be content I had to be a slut, but she always made me laugh. I didn't have time for men. Any dates I went on turned into disasters. I knew deep inside, however, that Iris was right. I wasn't going to have a full life all by myself.

A few weeks before, a friend had given me an antique Afghanistan prayer necklace, which had a small compartment in it that I assumed was meant to hold a little prayer. I decided to write a letter to God (whatever God meant; every day it changes for me). It went something like this:

> Dear God,
>
> Thank you for all you have given to me in life, and the way you have guided me. Please help me remain open to the lessons you have in store for me, so that I may follow my divine path and do what I am meant to do in life. Please keep me addiction-free, open, and always willing to learn and grow.
>
> If it is in the plan to meet a man, please have him be on a similar spiritual path, healthy, open, creative, honest, kind, funny, fun, adventurous, have good taste, and be happy. May he come from a good and kind family who have similar morals and values to mine. And please, make sure he has a job.
>
> I turn my will and my life over to you, and remain open.
>
>> Love,
> > Me

I rolled the little piece of paper up and slid it inside the necklace. I wore the necklace and ten days later, something magical happened, and after that, the necklace broke!

On this particular Saturday, I was coming down with a cold. I was in bed all day. Iris came and urged me to attend the art show. I didn't want to be a flake with my friends, so I rallied, picked up an Emergen-C vitamin mix and a bottle of water, and headed to the party. Going by myself didn't bother me at all—I was used to it. I meet people rather easily, and I'll talk to a mannequin.

I went to the party wearing a mini fur vest, which I got at an antique shop in Peru, a burnt orange skirt that I had made into a dress, and piles of my Pakistani and Afghan jewelry. The outfit was quintessentially me. Gypsified, if you will. As soon as I walked in, I saw a guy walking across the other end of the gallery who was dressed all in black. He had long dark hair, a dark beard, and a wide-brimmed, black hat. I was instantly transmitted in my mind to another century. I pictured this guy on a rolling library ladder in an old apothecary room, surrounded by taxidermy and maps. I was fascinated. I wanted to speak to this person who had aroused this connection in me. I wanted to ask him questions and learn from him. Don't ask me why. These are just the first thoughts that ran in my head when I saw him.

In addition to being attracted by his mysterious aura, the fact that he was drop-dead gorgeous might have also crossed my mind. But when he disappeared through the crowd I thought, *Oh well. He wasn't going to talk to me anyhow. Way too cool. And I am a total dork.*

I found my friend Francesco upstairs working the decks from a balcony and hung with him for a while. Then, out of absolutely nowhere, my mystery man looked up and waved to Fran.

As the wide-brimmed hat guy climbed the steps, I nearly pushed Francesco off the balcony with excitement.

"You know that guy!?" I asked. I made Fran promise to introduce me. "I have never felt so strongly about someone in my life," I said, nearly breathless. "I am smitten."

"Ally, I forgot his name," Fran said in a rather uninterested manner that didn't capture the electricity of the moment. "Just help me out when I introduce you."

I hastily applied some Chapstick (I don't care for lip gloss) and nervously started chewing on a cinnamon toothpick, which was my crutch for quitting smoking, which I did during the German protocol.

"Don't worry," I assured him. "I forget people's names all the time. I know what to do."

The man in the hat emerged from the stairs and our eyes met. I put out my hand and said, "Hi, I'm Alexandria. What's your name?"

"Steve. Nice to meet you."

A very tall guy had come upstairs with my mystery man, and he was rather intimidating. Anyone over six two is a little bit alarming to me. The tall friend of Steve's put out his hand and introduced himself. "Hi, I'm Eric."

Steve and I had a brief and funny conversation about cinnamon toothpicks. He had an uncle who made homemade cinnamon toothpicks back in the day. This delighted me. We had something in common.

Later we found each other again in the dense crowd of art folk. We spoke for a long while, as if no one else were around us in the gallery. It felt so natural and comfortable, like talking with an old friend (maybe from a past life?). A photographer approached and remarked, "You make a really adorable couple."

I played along and made up a random story just for fun. "We are not officially together, but last night I decided it would be fun to paint his whole body hot pink with a powdered paint pigment. He woke up in the morning shocked but intrigued!"

Spontaneous? Definitely. Kooky? Zany? Positively.

A few other people commented on the fact that we looked good together. It's one of those comments that both make you blush and get you all hot and red and sweaty and embarrassed. I couldn't deny that what they were saying was true. It didn't occur to me, however, that we would possibly go any further in any sort of romantic way. *There is no way this guy is single,* I thought.

I left him with my phone number and he gave me his, and we parted ways. I kept my expectations low. I thought he might be a new friend or perhaps we might work together in some capacity one day, or that my father and uncle would work with him. Steve was then the creative director at Warner Music Group, and my uncle Andy and my dad were involved with a lot of music and merchandising licensing deals with celebrities. There was a future with this guy. I just didn't know exactly what it was.

When I got home later that night, I saw a text from Steve. It said something like, "It was so lovely meeting such a wonderful woman... let's hang out this week." I had ended a relationship with an ex-boyfriend named Tim about a year before.

Over the previous months I had gone out on a few dates with different types of guys; some were setups and others were with guys I knew. After a while I became discouraged. I was just dating the wrong people, guys who were looking for the next cool thing or place to be. None of them seemed to want to commit on any level, let alone with someone who had all the baggage I had on my train car. So I decided to keep my expectations low with Steve.

The following week, we went out three times. The first night we were together was something of a spontaneous act out of loneliness on my part. We had set our first date for the following night, on Tuesday. But the Monday before I was going to an art show downtown and didn't feel like going alone. So I just called Steve to ask if he was available. We ended up spending most of the evening together.

Our first official date, on Tuesday night, he asked if I wanted to go see the Christmas windows at Bergdorf Goodman. I have to say, it was a good start on his part. It was exactly something that I liked to do. It was bitterly cold night, though, and I mean *frigid*. I wore this 1970s-era black print, silk chiffon dress with a big, frilly collar, billowy sleeves, and buttons down the front, but underneath it I wore two pairs of leggings: a pair of wool tights, and silky leggings over those so the dress wouldn't stick to the wool. I also wore two long-sleeved T-shirts under it, both low cut enough to match the neckline of the dress. I wore a brown suede and shearling aviator jacket from Ralph Lauren that I got for Christmas years before, which I never wore around my dad. I had on high, high-heeled booties and a wool hat and mittens.

After the windows, we ended up in a Japanese teahouse in Midtown, almost frozen stiff. We were at ease with each other instantly.

The third consecutive night he asked me to meet him and his friends at a bar in the Lower East Side. We ended up making our way to Don Hill's.

On the dance floor at the club, the song "Space Oddity" by David Bowie blared over the speakers. It was the perfect soundtrack for a first kiss. I felt as though I were floating in space. I couldn't even feel the pain from the six-inch, pony-skin stilettos I was wearing.

After Christmas, Steve went to Costa Rica with some friends for a surfing trip. He casually invited me to join him, not expecting that I would actually do it.

From Mustique, after our family Christmas, my brother Richard escorted me to meet up with Steve. There was no way he was going to let his big sister go alone to Costa Rica to meet up with some guy. I arrived with that same burnt orange skirt worn as a strapless dress, strappy sandals, and a huge black felt sunhat with lots of silver bracelets piled up on my little wrists.

When we landed, Steve, Richard, Eric (the tall intimidating friend), and I all went to lunch together. Once lunch was over, Richard 100 percent approved of this mystery guy and got on the next plane out. He knew I was in good hands.

I fell in love with Steve in the Monte Verde jungle of Costa Rica. We got lost in the rain, had two flat tires, were stranded, and had to stay in a random motel, and we had the time of our lives. We laughed so much my stomach hurt, but this time in a very good way.

I didn't want the trip to end and it seemed the universe didn't want it to end, either. As it happened, the northeastern United States was buried under a major snowstorm, and I was flying standby on JetBlue as it was, so there was no way we could fly into New York. Instead we got a flight to Miami for a connecting flight to Barbados. From Barbados we hopped on a plane to Mustique.

We spent New Year's on the island, where he met my entire family: my mom, her husband, my dad, his wife, her ex-husband and his girlfriend, all the kids, my aunt, my uncle, and their kids. It was nuts. If Steve could get through this, I thought, we really did have a shot.

When we got back to New York, the second of January 2011, we officially decided to date exclusively. Steve's parents and sister were in town waiting to see him for the New Year, and he followed my lead by inviting me to meet his family for dinner that evening. I was nervous as hell, and definitely not as calm, cool, and collected as Steve was meeting my family.

It seems completely mad that we met each other's families so quickly, but it just felt right, and we knew we were in it for the long haul that New Year's Eve. We just knew.

twenty-eight

EAST MEETS WEST AND CLOSES THE DOOR

*"I find hope in the darkest of days, and focus in
the brightest. I do not judge the universe."*
—DALAI LAMA

Here's something about Lyme disease you might not know: It hates happy endings.

If I had been on a roller coaster, I was finally at the tippy-top, loving every second, with NAHM and Steve and life in general. Steve's thirtieth birthday was approaching and I was planning a big two-part surprise party for him in New York. I had a lot of tasks at hand in the office and with the party.

One day I found myself at my desk at the NAHM office on Thirty-Ninth Street on the phone with three notepads and two laptops in front of me, trying to juggle about five different things at once. All at once, I had cartoon brain. Remember when the safe fell on Wile E. Coyote in the Road Runner cartoon and he wobbled around in circles with a whirling halo of Tweety birds? Yeah, that's the one. My brain just stopped working. I grabbed my coat and raced downstairs to get some air. I was hyperventilating. *This can't be happening*, I said to myself. *It can't be back, it can't be back.*

I knew that I had felt a little off, but I chalked it up to the stress of our last fashion show. I walked out of the building without a plan or destination. I came upon a church and walked in. It had been six years since the Christmas Eve at the church in Bedford Village where I fell on my knees and asked the priest to grant me sleep, and the memory of that night came flooding back. Here I was again, surrounded by stained glass and statues, at the end of my rope. This time, however, the church was nearly empty. There was the faint scent of incense in the air. I knelt in a pew with my face in my hands, the way my mother used to do, and prayed for help.

Just then, my phone buzzed. It was a text from Nary. "Where are you? Are you okay?"

"Not okay," I texted back. I wrote that I was in the church down the street.

By the time Nary arrived I was a mess, with mascara trails and hair stuck to my face. I couldn't stop shaking. I felt weak and limp. I could feel the hot blood pulsing through my veins and my joints swelling up like balloons. I had been feeling more rundown than usual the past couple of weeks but thought it was just because I was working so much. I thought the last treatment had taken away my symptoms for good and that I never ever would have to shut down again. I didn't continue following the German protocol after I was treated, for more than seven months. I became lazy, and work and life took over. My strict diet became more and more lenient. I didn't even take any drops to keep my toxicity low. I didn't think that I really had to because of how well I felt after the German treatment.

"It's going to be okay. Take as much time as you need," he said as he hugged me. "Just take care of yourself."

Those words, "Just take care of yourself," were overwhelming. How? How was I supposed to take care of myself if I thought I already was taking care of myself? What else could I do? *Do I have to be on treatments and diets and herbs for the rest of my life? Can't I just live and eat normally?* I was disappointed in myself, confused, frustrated, and I had no idea what to do with myself next.

After Nary left, I wandered through the Fashion District. I thought some air and some space would help. I was in a scene from a movie, the one where the heroine is on the verge of a nervous breakdown. I walked to Bryant Park. Big mistake. It was the first pretty springlike day of the year and it was a mob scene. I stood there frozen among what seemed like a million lives happening around me. I'd get a short glimpse of where I was and then my brain would turn off, as if someone were flipping a light switch.

I was sure I was going out of my mind.

I called Steve at his office. He said he would come home as quickly as possible.

"How could I have let this happen again?" I asked him.

I beat Steve back to the apartment and sat for a while by myself. My brain had cleared a little and I was able think through my situation. I had not let it happen to me again. It wasn't my fault. It was the fault of this fucking disease. I wasn't going crazy and I wasn't going to give up. I might be only five feet tall, and Lyme might be the undefeated champion, but I'd already gone eleven rounds with it and nothing was going to keep me in my corner when the bell rang for the twelfth.

The next few months were really, really rough. I crawled back to Manhattan Advanced Medicine to see Nurse Lisa and Dr. Mangan-aro. It turned out my body had built up a lot of toxicity. Also, when the body is stressed, when adrenals are shot, and the body has been attacked over the years in specific areas (in my case stomach, joints, and brain), the tissue holds the memory. They were shocked to see how toxic my body had become once again. They told me I needed to start at square one.

"So square one it is," I said.

I could barely lift up my body in the morning to use the restroom, let alone think about starting this whole thing over again. *There must be some lesson, something that I am missing.*

Dr. Manganaro recommended I see Sheila Bath. Sheila is incred-ibly intuitive and a past-life regression healer. When I finally got the courage to call her, I felt immediately at ease and knew that this was the right next step for me. This was a totally alternative approach to my fighting my disease, but I was open and ready to embrace it.

I knew again in my heart that there was a spiritual solution to my illness and Sheila opened the door for me.

She was like a supercharged, fast-track therapist with tangible and straightforward solutions and advice. No bullshit. She started me on daily writing exercises, which changed my life. The exercises were called Written Intentions and Focus Wheels, her adaptation of the Abraham-Hicks law of attraction process. Of course all of the treatments over the years had beaten back Lyme, attacking the nas-tiest of the nasty spirochetes and strengthening my body to fight. But this was different. This was bigger. This was like the mother of all armies. And simpler than anything I could have imagined.

One of the insights I gained through this process was that I had often used my sickness as a way to hide away from doing things

I didn't want to do or face. It wasn't that I could arrange when I got sick, but when I did I often used it as the perfect excuse. I also learned that beating myself up only delays the healing process. Dr. Shander made me stop calling it "my Lyme disease." I didn't own it, and I certainly didn't want it. Negative language lowers your defenses against the disease, she told me. Instead of owning the disease, Shander told me to say, "I am overcoming Lyme disease" and to call it "the" disease, not "my" disease.

Maybe most important, I learned that I needed to share my experience with others who suffer from Lyme so they don't have to feel so isolated in their struggles. I knew that was the only way I was going to get and stay better.

It was in that insight that the idea for this book was born.

Here's the thing about listening for the universe to tell you what to do, though. It's not as if it calls you on the phone or texts you. It can, and often does, talk to you through other people, but you have to remain open to the idea there is a power outside of you that wants you well. I know this might sound crazy, but all I can do is tell you what happened to me and let the chips fall where they may.

If you do remain open to the idea, however, the results are amazing. When I first met Nary, back when he hired me to style and cast his fashion show, he was the subject of a documentary being filmed called *Dressed*. Later on, after we started NAHM, I accompanied Nary to a couple of screenings of the film at colleges and such. We were sort of the happy ending of Nary's story and would answer questions during the Q&A after the screening. During this time, I became friendly with the film's producer, Maryanne Grisz, who also happened to be a Reiki master. When she found out about my Lyme history, she offered to perform Reiki healings on me, a technique of channeling energy into my body, which she did in my apartment on a few Saturdays. Those treatments were amazing.

One day when I was having a real anxiety attack, Maryanne came over with an Ayurveda remedy that contained, I think, buttermilk, ghee, cardamom, cinnamon, and a dash of maple syrup. It was like Valium. It was really wonderful.

Because of Maryanne, I became interested in Ayurvedic medicine and one night Steve and I watched a couple of documentaries about it. In the middle of the second documentary, Dr. Scott Gerson came on the screen. He was an American living in New York. I grabbed a pen and paper and scribbled his name in giant letters across the page. Something, in an odd way, felt very familiar about him. The next morning, I jumped out of bed and called Dr. Gerson's office (doctor No. 11).

The following week, Steve and I pulled up to a large rustic home in Brewster, New York. I was wearing a vintage Doors T-shirt, which I had thrown on in what I thought was one of those last-minute fashion decisions I make as I walk out the door. The universe, however, was speaking to me.

We sat in the living room, which doubled as the waiting room. It was bright and sunny, and it had a lovely and healthy energy. I was wiggling my legs like a little kid, I was so excited.

Dr. Gerson came out of his office wearing a long Indian collarless cotton blouse and white cotton pants and black clogs, and he looked just as he did in the documentary, with a long brown ponytail, friendly face, and kind blue eyes. He smiled as if he was genuinely pleased to see us and welcomed us into his examining room. We removed our shoes and walked into a big room with Oriental rugs and two large chairs, which looked as if they were made for royalty in the eighteenth century. In the end of the room stood a big brass Indian goddess statue in front of one of the four large bookshelves lining the room.

"You are wearing my very favorite band on your T-shirt," Dr. Gerson said with a big smile.

My heart leaped.

Dr. Gerson asked me for a brief synopsis of my history. I told him what my parents were like, how I was raised. I was very honest, and I became a bit emotional when discussing the pressure I felt I was under running a business. I didn't want to let anyone down, and I felt that I had no choice but to be very successful.

After I opened my heart to the doctor, with Steve sitting next to me holding my hand, Dr. Gerson invited me to sit on the floor with him beside the statue. He had me take some long deep breaths and told me to focus on something that brought me peace, and I chose the statue. She was a strong, powerful goddess. The doctor chanted and took my pulse from my wrists for a long while.

"You are not hopeless, Ally," he said. "Your body has definitely been through a lot and has a lot of healing to do, but I can tell that you are indeed able to get better and overcome this."

Dr. Gerson scheduled me to come to the five-day Pancha Karma and take some herbs beforehand. Pancha Karma is an Ayurvedic seasonal detox. He gave me lemon balm oil drops to put under my tongue two times a day to calm my nervous system. He put me on a special "Vata" diet. There are three *doshas,* or energies, in everybody's human body: Vata, Kapha, Pitta. Usually one is more out of balance than the rest. In my case it was the Vata, which represents air. An out-of-balance Vata can produce a great amount of anxiety.

A month or so later, during June's summer solstice and full moon, I packed up a little suitcase, and Steve dropped me off at the doctor's house to join a group of people I had never met in a five-day Pancha Karma.

When I arrived for the first day of this Pancha Karma, I had no idea how much this seasonal detox cleanse would change me. I experienced everything from heart palpitation flare-ups, to tears, anger, and low blood sugar attacks. I kept the faith no matter how low I got, and surrendered myself into the hands of the doctor and his protocol. In the morning, we had a light breakfast and would be given an enema created for each individual by the doctor, and wait to have our treatments. A woman would come fetch you and lead you to the steam room. After the steam, I was led into a room with a massage table and lots of sheets and hot oil. Two women would simultaneously massage in such a specific way to drain the lymphatic system and increase circulation. The doctor always met with the "herbalists" to prescribe what kind of massage and oil they should use. Some days I was given a Shirodhara treatment, which is a constant stream of hot oil being poured over your forehead for twenty minutes. This resets the nervous system as well. Some days I would be covered in clay and wrapped up in hot towels, which detoxed the body. Every day, Dr. Gerson would meet us for a healthy vegetarian Indian lunch. There were about eight people participating and living together undergoing these treatments tailor made for them and their ailments. There were people who had cancer, OCD, AIDS, or who just wanted to detox and feel healthy. It felt like I had checked myself into a rehab, but this time it was by choice and more relaxing.

Back home, I felt better than I had in a while. I think I really overcame a huge hurdle by doing the Pancha Karma. As good as the

German protocol was, I wanted to try something new "to make sure no rock went unturned." Always try something new, because you never know how it will help!

Steve and I were living temporarily at my dad's guest cottage in Greenwich, because it was calmer and the air was cleaner. I followed the Ayurvedic program thoroughly and felt so much clearer. But I was tired much of the time and struggling to keep NAHM afloat from my bed. I was also out of the loop on many design and business decisions, which was difficult for me. I was cracked wide open spiritually, and very vulnerable. When a NAHM employee came to my apartment back in New York one day to show me samples and sign some papers, I became a puddle of tears. I was so embarrassed about how weak I had become. I was feeling sorry for myself and felt defeated. Tangible and practical matters were hard for me to take seriously, and it was especially difficult to concentrate on anything due to the fact that all throughout July and August I had been suffering from bad headaches. For my body, I suppose Dr. Gerson's treatments could only go so far. I realize now that my body was trying to talk to me, well, yell at me. It was saying "STOP STRESSING YOURSELF OUT I CAN'T HANDLE IT ANYMORE!!!"

When late August rolled around, I knew I needed to get myself in gear to prepare our collection for the next fashion show in September. The *New York Times* wanted to do an article on us, and I needed the collection to be in tiptop shape. When I arrived at the new NAHM studio on Crosby Street in SoHo, the collection was not cohesive and nowhere near complete. I felt that I needed to rework the entire collection and start from scratch. Nary had a family emergency and had to be back in Ohio, and he had picked up the slack for me the past few months, so the least I could do was finish this collection to be presentable for New York Fashion Week and all of the pre-press.

I was able to make it into the office every day for half days. It was difficult for me to focus, and I felt drained after only two or three hours of working, but I was thrilled to be back and creative again. I insisted that my staff take care of themselves and take breaks often, eat healthy food, and recharge. I have always run a very organized and stress-free team, and I took pride in the fact that we were calm and organized, which is rare in the high-strung fashion world.

I was in the precarious position of having one foot in health and the other in Lyme, and although I never forgot how tentative my well-being was, there was a moment or two that I didn't want to believe my health was so fragile. One day I went out to eat with some of Steve's relatives who were in town. I knew that pizza was not on the Lyme diet plan, but I didn't want to seem like a picky eater. I was so thin that I didn't want anyone to judge me and think I was on some diet for vanity reasons. I just wanted to be normal and fit in.

I ate two pieces of delicious pizza and might have had a little bite of dessert. After the meal, Steve and I went to meet some friends. I was walking my bike beside him on the sidewalk. One minute Steve was asking me a question and the next thing I knew he was putting me in a cab to take me home. I couldn't remember my address or the code to my lock for the bike. It was as if I'd had a mini-seizure. The gluten, dairy, and sugar had inhibited my brain function. The stress I was under trying to get ready for Fashion Week didn't help.

That evening, I talked to Dr. Shander. "You know better than to eat crappy food," she said.

I got so mad I threw the phone. I was already angry with myself. I didn't need anyone else scolding me.

The next day I was standing in my kitchen making tea, and a burning hot yellow liquid began to leak out of my rear end. I know it's not the most attractive visual, but I'm telling you it was like acid. It was uncontrollable. I completely freaked out and sobbed out of helplessness and pure pain-panic.

I later learned that it was my gallbladder reacting to toxins. I went back to Dr. Manganaro immediately, and he said there was a possibility that they might have to remove my gallbladder. There were studies and cases claiming the IV antibiotic I had been on several years ago greatly damaged patients' gallbladders. I went on an aggressive series of homeopathies as well as a super-strict diet and cleanse, and it saved me from having surgery.

My gallbladder turned out to be the least of my worries.

It was three days before the *New York Times* writer was to come into the office. We were really making some good progress on the collection. I was beginning to be excited about ideas and fabrics and silhouettes and trims. Finally. Our staff was amazing. That they were pulling the collection together at all was a feat, but that they were going to make it happen on deadline was a miracle. During this time, my headaches were becoming more and more consistent, daily in fact. My father was concerned and wanted me to go to a migraine specialist, but I told him I was okay, I just had a lot on my plate and needed to focus.

I left the studio at 9 p.m. I had wanted to stay longer, but my staff took one look at me and sent me home. The over-the-counter migraine medication wasn't cutting it.

I woke up the next day with the same blinding headache that had now lasted more than twenty-four hours. I immediately called the migraine specialist my dad suggested. I went in to see Dr. Green at Mount Sinai Hospital. I walked into the office wearing dark sunglasses, like Jackie O. Dr. Green thoroughly examined me and interviewed me.

"I don't think your body does well with a lot of stress. You need to slow down and try to take it easy."

I responded defensively, "But I have a collection to show, and this company means everything to me. I can't ignore what I started and throw it all away."

"It's either your company or your health," he said with a small, knowing smile. "I am admitting you into the ER immediately for an IV and CAT scan, just as a precaution. We need to check this out and make sure it's nothing serious."

I called Steve to let him know what was going on. I didn't want to worry anyone, but just in case, I didn't want to be alone, either.

It turned out that I had a small aneurysm in my brain. Whether or not it was Lyme related I'm not sure. The migraines were Lyme related, though, and without them the doctor might not have done the CT scan and found the aneurism. It was too small to clamp in surgery. The only thing we could do was keep an eye on it. The migraine specialist had suggested that I might want to think about living somewhere a little calmer and cleaner than New York City.

I knew I needed to be on a totally different path, and for good.

Steve and I had been together for two and a half years at this point. He was ever patient and constantly loving. He was my number-one advocate and supporter next to my dad. Together they formed a kind of tag team to help me through this latest relapse. Steve called my dad to tell him what the doctor had found. Dad was adamant about one thing, and Steve agreed with him. On some level, I knew it was inevitable.

NAHM had to close, once and for all.

It was the right decision, but it was heartbreaking.

I wanted so much for everything to be normal, and each time "normal" seemed in my grasp, Lyme, or Lyme-related illnesses, would snatch it away from me.

Right after Christmas, Steve and I left for Mustique. We'd been talking about living on the island for some time. Steve was transitioning out of his office job at Warner Music Group and he was able to work for them remotely. I was still following the protocol from Dr. Gerson, and I did another Pancha Karma for the fall season. Even though I knew Ayurveda was working, I was not willing to take any chances. I had a feeling that there was one last doctor I needed to see. Don't ask me how or why I thought this, but my intuition knew there was still something else out there that would really be the very last home run, once and for all.

A few months earlier, in early November 2012, I heard about a new Lyme specialist who was supposed to be a genius and miracle worker. Dr. Stanley Kacherski would be the twelfth and last Lyme doctor I would see on my journey back to health. Kacherski is at the very top of the Lyme field. He was the first in his field to create his own homeopathies by using an infected tick. Three of the top homeopaths, from Germany, Switzerland, and India, had trained him. Based on basic homeopathic principles, that the body can heal itself, his treatment system was complex, but he led me step by step.

I began right away and started to feel the Herxheimer. Dr. Kacherski was smart to not tell me how many more cycles of the treatment I had to go through. I took all the treatments with me to Mustique. Every morning, I made fresh coconut milk shakes with pumpkin seed powder, celery, and parsley, with an apple to alkalize my system and lower any inflammation.

We worked out of "the black box," which was actually like a hard-cased, old-fashioned doctor's bag. It contained little glass vials with cork caps that were filled with teeny-tiny white pellets of magic that healed the psyche and the body to the deepest layers of my being. They reset the emotional subconscious, so to speak.

They came from a very prestigious homeopathic specialist in India. I know that they were very powerful—the treatment was intense and went beyond the physical plane. Our cells hold unhealthy negative memories and these pills would help release them. After taking them, I would experience severe anxiety and emotional weakness. I was told that I was mourning the loss of the disease I was letting go of, mourning for all the turmoil my body had gone through. It seemed to target where I was most vulnerable.

I wanted a family of my own. I had wanted to be a mother from my earliest memories. I was fearful that Steve would not want to be with someone who was so sensitive. I was fearful that I could never work the way I wanted to. This, too, I mourned.

When my emotions finally settled down, I felt a release I had never felt before from the bondage of a pain I had been living with for most of my life. The black box really rocked my world. It was as if I had placed my Lyme into the basket of a hot air balloon, gased and fired it up, and let it go.

I started to paint again—I hadn't had a paintbrush in my hand for three years. Steve and I set up an art studio in the guest cottage on the beach and painted together. It was incredible how much creativity poured out. I began a new series, which I now realize was symbolic of my healing.

I began doing daily meditations, which made me feel balanced and whole and centered. I call these *guided chakra meditations*.

We had friends come visit us in Mustique. We cooked every meal together every day and I painted. It was blissful. Steve did his work for Warner Music remotely, and we set up a little office in the dining room. We were like two old people in our seventies living the life of gypsies—a life of simplicity and happiness.

I volunteered at the local preschool, where I read to the local children and played games with them. Once a week, Steve and I also ran an after-school art class at the local elementary school. Being around children filled me with laughter and hope and perhaps awakened an instinct in me that had been buried under Lyme disease for a long time.

Every day I meditated and wrote my intentions and did a focus wheel on the beach in the back of our house. I wrote about moving to a house where it was warm and open and where Steve's and my relationship would grow stronger and stronger, and where creativity would flow.

Every day in the sun I felt better, and further from the shadow of Lyme.

twenty-nine
HIGHWAY TO HEAVEN

"The air was soft, the stars so fine, the promise of every cobbled alley so great, that I thought I was in a dream."
—JACK KEROUAC, *ON THE ROAD*

In the spring of 2013, Steve received a job offer on the West Coast. That June we packed my car and drove across the country. We chose the southern route and took our time. I was still taking treatments, so while Steve drove I would nap. One day I awakened as Steve was pulling into Dollywood, Dolly Parton's theme park in eastern Tennessee. "Surprise!" He smiled. We went on every ride there and I had so much fun.

Along the way to Los Angeles, we stayed in travel lodges and motels and ate at truck stops and diners, though I had to be careful with what I ordered—a burger wrapped in lettuce was one of my favored choices. We stopped at Graceland and ate famous barbecue in Memphis. We went to the Grand Canyon, the memory of which awes me still. We stayed in a dude ranch and spent two days in Las Vegas, where Steve met his work contact.

I was so excited to be in Vegas—it was my first time as an adult.

Steve and I stayed at the Mandalay Bay and that night went to the club in the hotel. Steve worked with the deejay who was performing. I played a little blackjack and won. By the second day I was nauseous from all the cigarette smoke and couldn't wait to leave!

Vegas aside, the road trip across the country was wonderful and just what the doctor ordered. I'd spent so many years battling my disease, and since so much of that time the battle took place on a spiritual plane, it was almost as if the universe was telling me to put my feet on the ground and feel the gravel of the road under my shoes.

"There's a big shiny world out there, Ally," it was saying. "Go take a look."

When we were in Mustique, I'd meditated and done focus wheels envisioning a place where Steve and I could live, a home that was warm, bright, and open. The thought of staying on Mustique never entered my mind. It was far too isolated and unrealistic for a young couple; we weren't running away from the world, we wanted to be part of it.

I'd also never considered living in Los Angeles. I am very trusting, and I always want to think the best of people. But I'm not naïve, at least not anymore. I've learned how to respect my instincts and follow my gut. I have a yellow, orange, and red flag system. Yellow means someone who is harmless—a little clingy but with kind intentions and a good heart. Orange means someone who is codependent and doesn't know they have ulterior motives. And red, well, it just means *Stay away*.

But then Steve got the call, and L.A. was where we were headed. I immediately called my brother Richard, who helped put my mind at ease. He'd been living on the west side of L.A. for a few years.

"It's so beautiful, Ally," he said. "I wake up every day happy."

We rented an old, Spanish-style house in Silver Lake, which is a bit more like New York in the creative sense of the word; maybe like the Williamsburg of L.A. The house was quaint and peaceful and surrounded by little fountains and beautiful foliage. It had a fireplace, plenty of outdoor space, and room for an art studio. I painted and cooked three meals a day.

In L.A. I met really good people: healthy, kind, creative, grounded. I struck up a friendship with a girl who ran a very cool vintage clothing store. There were none of those flighty L.A. people I'd always feared.

One day I decided to stop at Trader Joe's to pick up some things to cook for dinner for Steve and me. As I waited on the checkout line, I saw a package of chocolate-covered cherries, which are a guilty pleasure of mine. I knew I wasn't supposed to have them, but every once in while you just have to throw caution to the wind.

I opened the package and began eating them in line. As I got to the parking lot, a car came to a screeching halt in front of me and out of it climbed two West Hollywood boys in tight jean shorts and mesh tank tops.

"Are you Ally Hilfiger?" one asked almost breathlessly. I nodded. "Oh my God, we are such big fans of *Rich Girls*!" Every now and again someone would recognize me from the show, and I guess it had a second life as a cult favorite, especially in the gay community. Still, I was always a little shocked by the mention of the show— it was really a different lifetime for me.

To be honest, I was a little flattered. They fawned over me and asked to take a couple of photos, which I was happy to do. As I got into my car, I was feeling really pretty good about myself. Then I looked in the mirror and saw I had chocolate all over my lips and chin!

* * *

Every day I thanked the focus wheels for how easy the move and transition were. I wrote my intentions on our road trip and kept a positive attitude. I was feeling really well. Although the treatments from Dr. Kacherski were tedious and required patience and discipline, I was willing to do whatever it took, and whatever it took was working.

Years of antibiotics had destroyed my insides, though they had been extremely helpful treatments at the time. Now I kept things slow and steady when I felt well, and rested for a whole day after I traveled anywhere. I wasn't afraid to say no when asked to do one too many things. The days of spreading myself thin were over. I was wise enough to know when I needed to rest and take a nap and trained myself not to feel guilty for doing so. Los Angeles was so chill, and so far from the pressure in New York that had made me ill, that I knew I'd made the correct decision in moving there. Am I perfect at all of this? Absolutely not. If I'm at an Italian restaurant and I want to eat a bowl of rigatoni Bolognese, I'm going to. With that said, I try to follow an anti-inflammatory, immune-strengthening diet as best as I can.

It had been nearly ten years since I was diagnosed with Lyme disease. In that time I had created a toolbox for myself and filled it with spiritual and physical methods to help me get through anything my disease threw at me. The tools included phone numbers of healthy people, breathing exercises, writing practices, therapists, foods, herbs, meditation, and not lying to myself about when I didn't feel great.

After ten long years, I had developed a healthy sense of what really matters in life and what has meaning.

After ten long years, I finally had the clarity to know what I needed to be happy.

Dr. Shander had recommended someone named Joe Wilson, who taught me about powerful meditations. I did these special meditations and I imagined visiting with everyone in my life who had seen me through this torturous road with my health. In my meditation, I saw and told every one of my doctors, from Dr. Phillips to Dr. Kacherski, that I was better. I saw myself with Dr. Shander in her office, where I told her that I was completely healed. I transported myself to my backyard in Greenwich and told all my friends that I had been cured and didn't have a trace of Lyme left in my body. I saw Steve in our old apartment; Jaimie was there, too. I saw Uncle Billy in the attic on Round Hill Road and my island family on the beach in Mustique.

I swam in the healing ocean in Mustique with my mother, and she and I cried with happiness that I was free from Lyme. I fell into my father's arms and thanked him for all he had done, because he'd been so strong for me and it had all worked. In my imagination, the reactions on my parents' faces felt so real and true and beautiful.

Then I was able to see myself in the moment with all of my senses engaged, telling people I was totally healed, and I was. I remember feeling heat run through my body. It was as if I were injected with light that I imagined dissipating any dead or sleeping spirochetes.

As I opened my eyes, I kept that feeling I had experienced in my meditation. That feeling of being able to tell people I was healed, and feeling truly healed, once and for all. I think between the years of antibiotics, homeopathic treatments, detox diets, herbs, meditations, letting go of stress, and being in love, attempting to gain balance and happiness within myself might have seeped into my subconscious somehow. I felt healed. Maybe I would have to go through a few things here or there, but never would I ever have to be in fetal positions sobbing in agony, pain, confusion, or any other extreme symptoms of Lyme disease. I had filled a huge toolbox for myself over the past twenty-two years, to help me manage this illness. Though I know I am not 100 percent cured, you never are from Lyme disease, I feel healed in many ways. I feel stronger and more capable, and able to be honest when my stomach, brain, or joints flare up. It doesn't have to pull me into the pits of hell.

thirty

NOT AT ALL WHAT I WAS EXPECTING...

There is a moment in any journey where you look back and realize that it all finally makes sense. All of the treatments I'd taken, all of the setbacks, disappointments, and Lyme relapses I had experienced had not, in fact, been slides backward but necessary steps forward. The realization that the only way out of my sickness was through it was pretty sweet. In fact, I thought nothing could be more miraculous.

I was wrong.

Ten months after settling into our new home and life in Los Angeles, including my boyfriend's new job as creative director with a cool independent electronic label and a big-name artist, Steve was scheduled for a work trip to Japan with his whole team and I was invited. My mom had often told me about being pregnant with me and designing her women's sportswear collection in Japan. When I told her I was going on the trip she didn't offer any sightseeing advice; all she said was, "Don't eat the rattlesnake soup."

We landed in Kyoto, where we saw the Kinkaku-ji, the golden Buddhist temple, and a real geisha walking on the street. The following day we took the fast train to Tokyo. When people asked if I'd ever been there before, I'd say yes, but that I had been in my mother's abdomen at the time. We ate sushi for breakfast and felt like teenagers out on the town. There was an electric energy in the air with everyone on this Japan trip; it was tangible and delightful. I danced, ate, made love, laughed, ran, skipped, sang, and explored.

One month after Japan, Steve and I went to Santa Barbara, California, where I did two visual meditations. The morning meditation, which I did on the beach, was focused on creativity. Right after the meditation we saw dolphins jumping and swimming in the ocean in front of us. Later that day, we went to the house where Steve was born. It might have been a coincidence that my astrology chart had sent me to the place of Steve's birth, or maybe not.

The second meditation, to be done in the evening, was centered on my health. Through the magic of Google Maps, Steve found a lovely park with a bench where I could sit. My boyfriend stayed in the car, did a little meditation of his own, and watched over me to make sure there weren't any creeps around. I told him to visualize white light and sparkles swimming through my body. He was sweet and went along with my silly request. As I fell into the meditation, I went around to all the people I knew and loved and told them I was completely healed and cured. This time my imagination, however, threw in a little twist: While visiting all these people I saw myself pregnant.

In the meditation, my friends and family asked if the Lyme was affecting the pregnancy. No, I assured them. I told them that I had never felt better in my life, that I was totally cured, and that I felt absolutely amazing.

I remember being curious as to why the meditation would interpret me as pregnant. With all my body had been through, I wasn't even sure I could get pregnant. Steve and I had discussed the possibility and decided we would to try in a year or two. We had wanted some time just to feel healthy and free. To be honest, I didn't spend much time thinking about it. I just figured my meditation and imagination were projecting into the future. It wasn't until the next evening that it all made sense.

On our way back from Santa Barbara, we stopped in to see my mother, who had also moved to L.A., to be close to my brother and me. I had a few presents I'd found for her at an antique shop. As Mom and I were chatting, I lifted up my shirt and asked her if she thought I had gained a few pounds; I was feeling heavier than normal. She was politely honest, as usual, and said, "Yup, you don't look like yourself."

It was at that point when the possibility dawned on me. Steve, my mom, and I walked to the pharmacy, where I bought three pregnancy tests (and Steve bought a six-pack of Pabst Blue Ribbon beer). We rushed back to her house and I peed on all three sticks. A few minutes later, all of us crammed into the bathroom. My heart was racing.

All three tests were positive.

I don't know if it was right then, but if it wasn't it was soon thereafter that I found myself in the bathroom crying. The tears that streaked my face were different than the tears of years gone by, the tears of frustration and pain, the tears of hopelessness that chronic Lyme sufferers experience. Gone from my reflection was any trace of the doctors, the treatment, and the relapses. In their place was a new woman, a pregnant woman, crying tears of joy. Don't get me wrong, it's not like the Lyme disease has completely disappeared. I still experience joint pain, nausea, memory loss, and other symptoms of Lyme, and I probably always will. But I'm different now and the realization of that is truly a miracle, and a moment I wish for for everyone who suffers from Lyme disease. Even in the most chronic cases of Lyme like mine, hope is the most powerful antidote.

epilogue

I began writing this book in 2012. It grew out of my daily writing exercises and focus wheels in which I had announced to the universe my intention to help others with Lyme disease. Over the last few years, I've become more involved with the Global Lyme Alliance, serving on its board of directors. Last year, along with Yolanda Foster and Latin singing star Thalia, I was honored with the Courage Award at the Global Lyme Alliance's annual gala in New York City. It was a night that glittered with celebrities and the brightest lights in the world of fashion. The most brilliant part of the evening, however, was the fact that we raised more than $3 million.

When I accepted my award, I told the audience a bit about my story and then asked them to focus on the youngest victims of Lyme disease. They are our daughters, sons, and grandchildren. Our future generation needs our help so they won't have to go through life in a fog and with chronic pain. Children ages three to fourteen are at the greatest risk at contracting the disease.

Our beautiful, healthy daughter, Harley Elizabeth Hilfiger Hash, was born on February 8, 2015 at Cedars-Sinai Medical Center in Los Angeles. Steve brought an iPod so there'd be music in the room. When I was trying to push, the doctor told Steve to change it to something a little more upbeat than Native American flute music. So Steve went to the iPod and pressed "shuffle" on the rock-and-roll playlist. My daughter came into the world to David Bowie's "Space Oddity," our song. She is the light of our lives and the motivation behind all that we do. Yet, Harley came into a world that still hasn't caught up to the ravages of Lyme disease. Countless numbers of Lyme sufferers continue to be undiagnosed or misdiagnosed, and many simply cannot afford the treatment.

This has to stop.

It has to stop now.

It can begin to stop with those lucky enough to not have Lyme disease. They are the ones who can turn the tide simply by keeping their hearts and minds open to those who do have the disease. We need your help and support. We need you to fight for us.

We need you to believe us.

For all of us with Lyme disease, having hope and allowing in the positive energy of the universe gives us a fighting chance. I know I was in a unique position to be able to see many different doctors, and seek out some crazy treatments, but that was purely my experience. It doesn't have to be yours. Many people do not become as sick as I did, nor do they have the resources to try almost every treatment under the sun. I realize this, and I hope no one has to go through as many relapses. I also hope that this story has offered some laughter, clarity, and awareness. If my book brought you a glimmer of hope then it has served its purpose. Above all, whether you've suffered from Lyme for twenty days or twenty years, I hope you find your silver lining as I did.

Thank you for reading, and may love be with you always.

appendix one
TWO DOCTOR'S OPINIONS

DR. HARRIET KOTSORIS

Chief Science Officer, Global Lyme Alliance

Chronic Lyme statistics should both surprise and shock you. There are probably 350,000 new cases of Lyme disease per year, and researchers, ones from esteemed institutions, have found that even when antibiotics are given in a timely fashion and in standard doses, 20 to 30 percent of those will fail conventional treatment and go on to develop a very disabling and chronic Lyme disease. By those metrics, there are up to 100,000 new people suffering from chronic Lyme disease each year. Add it all up over the last thirty years or so since the causative bacterium of the illness, *Borrelia burgdorferi,* was identified, and there are 3–4 million chronic Lyme sufferers alive today, people for whom we have no diagnostic markers or treatment options of major success.

How disabling can chronic Lyme get? Well, it's a spectrum. In the best of a bad circumstance, there are some who have ups and downs and can be functional on some days and on some days can't do a thing. In the worst, you have chronic Lyme sufferers who have the functional ability of a class 4 congestive heart failure patient or a person who can sit in a wheelchair and do practically nothing else.

Unfortunately, Lyme disease is a politically and scientifically charged problem. For many years, the Infectious Diseases Society of America, and a lot of physicians out there, felt Lyme was easy to diagnose and easy to cure. As time went on, science, and I think mainstream science, has shown that this is not the case. Even in the best of hands, diagnostic tests today are only reliable about half the time; as much as 50 percent of the results can be false negatives. Even those diagnosed can face daunting odds of full recovery.

Patients on the standard antibiotic treatment of doxycycline for four weeks, or even ones on an intravenous of ceftriaxone or Rocephin for three to four weeks, will fail treatment 20 to 30 percent of the time. Why? We're still not completely sure. We do know that some of the failures are due to delay in the original diagnosis and treatment, but many scientists believe that it is a result of a post-treatment immunological component. In other words, some people develop an autoimmune type of response to the infection that cannot be reversed because, in the face of antibiotics, this devious bacterium goes dormant and hides. When the infection reactivates at a later date, it wreaks havoc on the body and its immune system so that patients can look as if they have lupus, rheumatoid arthritis, and the like. When the nervous system gets involved, patients can also look as if they have Parkinson's, multiple sclerosis, and even Lou Gehrig's disease. What triggers the reactivation? Stress, seasonal change, surgery, sleep deprivation, another illness, you name it. Lyme is not unique in this regard. There are a lot of bacteria that behave in the same way: tuberculosis, *E. coli,* syphilis. The list goes on. How to eradicate these persistent infections is one of the major problems in the infectious diseases world today. They're tough. There isn't an easy answer.

Many medical breakthroughs are often born out of controversy and division. Perhaps a cure for Lyme will come in the same manner. We can hope. We do know the stakes are high in that a cure for Lyme might actually have applicability to other diseases as well. If we crack this, we might be able not only to help the millions upon millions who suffer from the debilitation of chronic Lyme, but to solve a slew of other problems in the process.

Those of us working on the front lines of the Lyme epidemic are not a fringe element. We are not out there fighting for awareness just for the sake of fighting. This is a critically important problem, and it has scientific merit to it.

DR. ELLYN SHANDER M.D.

Throughout history great breakthroughs have come through awareness. Louis Pasteur saw microbes in a sea of bacterial ignorance. Scoffers of Isaac Newton finally saw the laws of gravity in flashes of brilliance. Courageous explorers sailed off in the face of "the world is flat" doubters and opened closed minds of Europe by sailing back with riches and wisdom. Now it is our time for science to wake up. We have the opportunity to fight and eradicate a scourge on our planet. We can save hundreds of thousands of people suffering lives crippled by pain and loss. But healing only happens with awareness. The controversy over Lyme disease, with some even questioning its existence, is staggering. It is time that we emerge from the darkness of ambiguity and step firmly into identifying Lyme, and its co-infections, with predictable blood tests and no false negatives. It is time that we step into early detection and aggressive treatments. It is time to fully understand the vector of Lyme and how it hitchhikes on ticks. It is time for doctors and health-care professionals to educate themselves about acute Lyme disease, chronic Lyme disease, and the necessity for long-term treatments. It is time to mount a war against Lyme disease and make it a disease of the past.

Lyme disease has been called the "great imitator" in the psychiatric and medical literature. When it is manifested in a person, its chameleon presentation looks like many other diseases.

I became an "expert" on Lyme, out of necessity. For more than twenty-five years, patients have come to my office with some combination of symptoms of anxiety, mood changes, memory problems, personality changes, paranoia, nightmares, anxiety with air hunger, thought disorders, hallucinations, joint pain, muscle aches, headaches, vision problems, unsteady walking problems, flulike symptoms, and nerve pain. Energetic bright people are brought to their knees with an inability to think and function. They are besieged by rages and unexplained emotional surges. Teens change from being good students to being depressed and irritable, often with severe personality changes. People with Lyme often have had pets that went outside, or have walked in the woods, or simply lay on the grass on a sunny day. When asked if they had been tested for Lyme, most have said, "I don't have Lyme, my doctor sent a blood test . . ." Unfortunately the regular labs do not find Lyme with their present tests. Also unfortunately, despite an epidemic in our country, doctors are not thinking Lyme and pursuing this diagnosis. So these patients have worsening Lyme symptoms, and are often disabled by the time I see them, with no accurate diagnosis of a Lyme infection that was treated. I cannot stress loud enough that Lyme can be diagnosed clinically, the old-fashioned way. Yes, it is better to have a blood test from the more definitive labs, but if it looks like Lyme, smells like Lyme, and acts like Lyme, the early initiation of antibiotic therapy is crucial. Chronic Lyme takes a huge toll on the immune and neurological systems. One of my biggest joys is to make an accurate diagnosis and shepherd that person to specialized Lyme treatment. I have seen hundreds of patients who, like Ally, have endured a life of pain, confusion, and psychiatric symptoms. A life being robbed of its life force. We have an obligation to diagnose and recognize Lyme, leading to treatment and recovery.

It has been my privilege to diagnose, assist, support, and witness Ally's transformation on her journey to heal Lyme disease.

Ally's honest and openhearted writing of the impact of Lyme on her life is both horrifying and uplifting. Her fight back to health is awe inspiring.

The power of Ally's story is that it has so many levels of healing. Her poignant description of growing up with Lyme is heartbreaking. Undetection and no treatment left her an undefended and vulnerable eight-year-old unable to read or focus. Unlike healthy children who wake up with energy, she woke up exhausted, with little motivation, painful joints, and constant confusion in school. She was a child faced with a world she couldn't figure out, and no language to express the inner world of torture. Her years in schools, with diagnoses of learning difficulties and ADD, are common tangents for professionals who can't see Lyme disease. As her physical health deteriorated, we see her terrifying descent into hell. She gradually became unhinged with the addition of pot and alcohol, self-medicating her brain and body, inhabited by the enemy.

As we read her story, the next level becomes apparent. Her emotional journey is a personal story of transitioning from a young girl, privileged and immature, to a woman of self-discovery and maturity. Her gradual awakening to her own abilities, her own opinions, and her own choices was a joy to help shepherd. We see her begin to trust her own inner system, make her mistakes, but consistently walk toward health and self-care, navigating schedules of endless herbs, homeopathy, and antibiotics. Her sobriety, healthy diets, and avoidance of stress came from an inner commitment that this disease would not defeat her. Her warrioress emerged, determined to " climb mountains, forge rivers, and walk through rings of fire."

Thus begins her next level of healing, her spiritual journey, from victim to self-healer. It is difficult to do justice to the extraordinary privilege it has been working, guiding, and loving her on this journey. Her courage on her path of transformation has been extraordinary. Like a plant that turns its leaves to the light despite the obstacles, she has continually heartened me with her determination to find and nourish her inner light. We met sharing Ganesha, the elephant god, who overcomes all obstacles. And over the last ten years Ally has never wavered in looking for more spiritual connections. Healing happens with a connection to spirit, however one defines it. And she has a connection that is powerful and nourishing.

The great masters have said that facing adversity leads to our greatest growth, and that grief and suffering is the ultimate refining of the soul. Nobody chooses Lyme disease. Nobody chooses chronic suffering as they get better. But Lyme disease presents a rare opportunity to find our inner strength, our inner warrior, and our connection to spirit with a deep reverence for life and happiness. Fighting for health and stability, day after day, despite pain and confusion, illuminates our greatest warriors.

Ally stepped up to this challenge and to her next level of healing. Transformation happens with initiation, and then discovering one's own sovereignty through the journey. During our work together, I called her Princess Alexandria. I said we would work on her becoming a queen. We worked on her becoming aligned with her greatest goals and becoming an independent person committed to helping others for the greater good.

I watched Ally bloom over the years into the fighter that she is today. She evolved spiritually, recognized her own inner power, and overcame brain fog when it threatened to demolish her meditations and daily functioning. Ally followed and manifested her dreams. She is a joy to spend time with. Her appreciation of her life is grounded in almost losing her life to one of this planet's worst plagues. It is difficult to have a happy ending to an unhappy journey, but she punctuated her journey with happiness, hope, and laughter. Despite her suffering, she had faith during the darkness. She had courage in times of fear. And best of all, she had confidence that there was a rainbow at the end of her journey. Now when I spend time with Ally, her partner, Steve, and their little girl, Harley, I am filled again with the wonder of our human potential. Whatever the adversity we face as humans, we can overcome it.

Ally, it gives me great pleasure to call you Queen Alexandria. With great determination and courage you have arrived. Congratulations on your recovery, your persistence, and your transformation. You are a true pioneer.

May all your days be blessed with happy moments, good health, and love.

appendix two
FOCUS WHEELS AND WRITTEN INTENTIONS

Focus wheels and written intentions are among the most powerful spiritual tools I've come across—promise. This is an important secret to overcoming Lyme disease. It doesn't cost any money, doesn't involve doctors' offices, or needles, or pills, or anything like that. All it takes is a little bit of time, a little bit of faith, and a pad and pencil.

The focus wheel I use is based on the Abraham-Hicks law of attraction process.

Get a notebook and get those pencils sharpened. Come on! Get up and get them. Well, at least pay close attention. There are two different formulas. I'll start with the focus wheel first.

On the top of the page, write today's date. Next, write: "I AM SO GRATEFUL FOR EVERYONE AND EVERYTHING IN MY LIFE!!!"

Then, "I am so grateful to [the universe, God, higher power, the ocean, energy, a doorknob—whatever floats your boat]."

Then write: "Today is the best day in my life so far and it is so" (or if you want to focus on the whole year, or the upcoming week or month, then you write the previous statement accordingly).

Are you following me so far?

Here is when it gets wacky: Draw a circle in the middle of the page. Not a huge one, but like the size of the bottom of a water bottle. Inside the circle, write the following: and just ignore the language if it bothers you; just suck it up and write it. You can get over it if it bothers you.

"I LOVE EVERYONE AND EVERYONE LOVES ME. I BLESS EVERYONE AND EVERYONE BLESSES ME. I FORGIVE EVERYONE AND EVERYONE FORGIVES ME."

Got it? Not too hard, right? Okay, next, draw lines coming off the circle. Twelve lines. I like to call them sunbursts. In between each sunburst there will be room to write.

The reason why this thing is called a "focus wheel" is that you are going to choose a topic to focus on. It can be anything from health and recovery from Lyme disease, to body image and self-esteem, to buying and moving into a new home, to finding a partner to complete your life. Or a job you want! This stuff works, I am telling you honestly from the bottom of my heart.

I did plenty of focus wheels on my health and Lyme, but I'll use a more tangible example. Say you're moving into a new place; in each "sunburst" you might write the following:

I love it when . . . [e.g., my home is always safe and easy to deal with]

I love that . . . [e.g., moving into our new house was easy, went smoothly, affordable, and fun, with helpful, honest, kind, strong, organized people to help me do it]

I love it when . . . [e.g., my monthly expenses for my new home are lower than I expected and that I can always afford everything for my home]

I love that . . . [e.g., my home is always safe and protected and clean]

I love it when . . . [e.g., people always feel very comfortable and welcome and happy in our new home).

I love that . . . [e.g., my children are always safe, happy, healthy and protected in our new home, and that they thoroughly enjoy every aspect of our safe wonderful home. It is a perfect environment for them to grow up in).

I think you are starting to understand. Now, these statements are in present tense (even if you have not found that new home yet, or not acquired that job or found that perfect man). You have to pretend a little, and ALWAYS STAY IN THE POSITIVE. Language like "I love it when my boyfriend doesn't cheat on me" or "I love that our house isn't going to get robbed and burn down" is considered negative language. You have to figure out how to turn those things into positives. Like "I love that my boyfriend is a faithful respectful man who loves me unconditionally." Or "I love it when our home is always safe and protected by everything and everyone." Get it? Got it? GOOD!!

The next exercise is one that is really fun because you can just go on and on and put in as many details as humanly possible, which for these, is important to do. The more details, the more specific you can be, the better.

This next written formula is called "Written Intentions."

Get that notebook back out and go to a fresh page.

At the top of the page, write the date.

Next, you will write five (or more if you're feeling happy) things you are grateful for.

Example:

I am SO GRATEFUL for:
   1. My family
   2. My health
   3. My home
   4. Having love surrounding me always
   5. My dog
   6. My close and supportive friends

Now is the fun part. You have five intentions to create for your life. Anything your heart desires—reach for the stars! Sometimes this seems silly, or ridiculous, especially if you are feeling blue, but if you force your pen to the page and get out of yourself a bit, your whole mood will transform before your very eyes. It's very likely that you will become healthier and more vibrant on even a molecular level as well. It has been proven.

After you write what you are grateful for:

   1. I INTEND AND CREATE NOW . . . [e.g., that the home that we find is under our budget, airy, light, clean, safe for the children, private, beautiful, will fit all of our furniture and belongings, feels calm and peaceful. May our new home be white with blue shutters, and have land to have a garden big enough to grow seven different types of vegetables and fruit, too. May the soil be rich and healthy. There is enough room for our family vehicles. My family and I are always healthy and happy within the home and property]
   2. I INTEND AND CREATE NOW . . . [e.g., that the man of my dreams is available, single, taller than I, has a job, a good

honest family with good morals and values, funny, adventurous, fun to be around, creative, easy to talk to, gets along with all of my friends and family, is supportive, compassionate, empathetic, understanding, on the same wavelength as I am, very handsome, amazing in bed, has perfect chemistry with me, has great taste that is on par with my own, has his goals in a similar direction as I, lives near me, has healthy feelings toward being committed and wanting a family, is very healthy physically, mentally, spiritually, and emotionally]

3. I INTEND AND CREATE NOW . . . [e.g., that I feel healthy and productive]
4. I INTEND AND CREATE NOW . . . [e.g., accomplishing all that I set out to do today and feel great for it]
5. I INTEND AND CREATE NOW . . . [I think you've gotten the idea!]

And that's it! Now close your notebook and go about your day. See what happens. See what your mind-set is like. Now wake up and do it all again tomorrow. In the words of Larry David, it's pretty, pretty, pretty cool.

For more information, or to donate for a Lyme-free world, please visit: www.globallymealliance.org.

To prevent you, your children, and your pets from getting bitten by a tick, buy this wonderful organic insect repellent at www.ticktocknaturals.com.

NOTES

1 http://www.ncbi.nlm.nhi.gov/pubmed/7943444.

2 http://underourskin.com/news/lyme-destroys-families-update-jordan-fisher-smith.

3 Polly Murray, *The Widening Circle: A Lyme Disease Pioneer Tells Her Story* (New York: St. Martin's Press, 1996).

4 http://annals.org/article.aspx?articleid=691188.

5 http://www.lymeresearchalliance.org/test-diagnostic.html.

6 http://www.ncbi.nlm.nih.gov/pmc/articles/PMC3547183/.

7 http://www.lymebook.com/chronic-lyme-symptoms.

8 http://www.mentalhealthandillness.com/Articles/LymeDiseaseAndCognitiveImpairments.htm.

9 http://www.ilads.org.

10 http://new.homelesschildrenamerica.org/mediadocs/280.pdf.

11 http://www.northeastern.edu/news/2015/06/researchers-discovery-may-explain-difficulty-in-treating-lyme-disease/.

12 http://www.merriam-webster.com/medical/Jarisch–Herxheimer%20reaction.

13 https://chronicillnessrecovery.org/index.php?option=com_content&view=article&id=161.

14 http://www.cdc.gov/lyme/treatment/.

15 http://www.cdc.gov/lyme/stats/.

ACKNOWLEDGMENTS

A project like this one would not exist without the help of many. First and foremost, I would like to thank my soulmate and best friend—father of our daughter, Harley—Steve Hash. You have been a source of constant encouragement, inspiration and true love. You are my safe harbor.

I also wouldn't have known how to navigate the seas of my life, let alone the choppy waters of telling my story, without the unconditional and unwavering love from my parents, Tommy and Susie. You inspired me to be my own person. Thank you to my brother Richard, sisters Elizabeth and Kathleen, Dee and little Sebastian, I love you to the moon and back. I would also like to thank the wonderful Hash family. A special thank you to Roberta Sorvino and Celsa Avendano, my honorary family. I would have to extend this section five more pages if I were to list out all of my loving and wonderful friends who are my inspiration, cheerleaders, and folks who made me laugh amist moments of doubt or stress.

Special thank you needs to go to Yolanda Foster, not only for her support in our mutual battle against Lyme, but for introducing me to the best literary agents ever: Jan Miller and Lacy Lalene Lynch of Dupree/Miller. You are angels on earth and a dream team. I'll be eternally grateful to Rolf Zettersten and Kate Hartson from Hachette. Thank you for trusting in this memoir and for the help from your whole publishing team: Patsy Jones, Andrea Glickson, Katie Broaddus, Alexa Smail and everyone else at Hachette who participated in the making of this book. I would also like to thank my wonderful PR team at PMK, Lauren Auslander and Jennifer Abel. You girls are dynamite! And thanks to Dan and Marc for leading me to you!

There were times in the beginning when the process felt overwhelming. So thank you Jeanne Darst for showing up at my house every Wednesday at 1pm to read a new chapter. You helped guide me over the first hurdle of writing my story honestly and fearlessly. Brian McDonald, thank you for guiding me through structuring, rewriting and filling in the missing parts. I am forever grateful for your knowledge, friendship and hard work.

I am also very grateful for my father, Dr. Harriet Kostorsis, and Dr. Ellyn Shander for the contributions you worked on so diligently. They were very helpful for this book.

Finally, I'd like to thank the many doctors and healers who have helped me and Global Lyme Alliance for tirelessly searching for a cure. Without you I would never have been able to build my bridge back to life, let alone write this book! Thank you, from the bottom of my heart.

ABOUT THE AUTHOR

ALLY HILFIGER is an artist, designer, and the daughter of fashion mogul and entrepreneur Tommy Hilfiger. She created, produced, and starred in *Rich Girls* for MTV, spearheaded the women's clothing line NAHM, and sits on the board of the Global Lyme Alliance and Project Lyme. She currently lives in Los Angeles with her husband, Steve Hash, and daughter, Harley. www.allyhilfiger.com.